Handbook for the Care of the Older Adult With Cancer

Edited by

Ann Schmidt Luggen, PhD, RN, CS, CNAA, ARNP

Sue E. Meiner, EdD, RN, CS, GNP

Oncology Nursing Press, Inc.
A subsidiary of the Oncology Nursing Society
Pittsburgh, PA

Oncology Nursing Press, Inc.

Publisher: Leonard Mafrica, MBA, CAE
Technical Publications Editor: Barbara Sigler, RN, MNEd
Staff Editor: Lisa M. George, BA
Creative Services Assistants: Chad Chronick, Dany Sjoen

Handbook for the Care of the Older Adult With Cancer

Library of Congress Card Number: 00-101135

ISBN 1-890504-16-5

Publisher's Note

This book is published by the Oncology Nursing Press, Inc. (ONP). ONP neither represents nor guarantees that the practices described herein will, if followed, ensure safe and effective patient care. The recommendations contained in this book reflect ONP's judgment regarding the state of general knowledge and practice in the field as of the date of publication. The recommendations may not be appropriate for use in all circumstances. Those who use this book should make their own determinations regarding specific safe and appropriate patient-care practices, taking into account the personnel, equipment, and practices available at the hospital or other facility at which they are located. The author and publisher cannot be held responsible for any liability incurred as a consequence from the use or application of any of the contents of this book. Figures and tables are used as examples only. They are not meant to be all-inclusive, nor do they represent endorsement of any institution by the Oncology Nursing Society (ONS). Mention of specific products and opinions related to those products do not indicate or imply endorsement by ONS or ONP.

ONS and ONP publications are originally published in English. Permission has been granted by the ONS Board of Directors for foreign translation. (Individual tables and figures that are reprinted or adapted require additional permission from the original source.) However, because translations from English may not always be accurate and precise, ONS and ONP disclaim any responsibility for inaccurate translations. Readers relying on precise information should check the original English version.

Printed in the United States of America

Oncology Nursing Press, Inc.
A subsidiary of the Oncology Nursing Society

Contributors

Ann Schmidt Luggen, PhD, RN, CS, CNAA, ARNP
President
National Gerontological Nursing Association
Professor of Nursing
Northern Kentucky University
Highland Heights, Kentucky
Chapter 1. Demographic Data: Cancer in Older Adults
Chapter 5. Nursing Care of the Older Adult With Lung
  Cancer
Chapter 9. Cancer Pain in the Older Adult

Sue E. Meiner, EdD, RN, CS, GNP
Research Patient Coordinator/Gerontologist/Nurse
  Practitioner
Washington University School of Medicine—Division
  of Geriatrics/Gerontology
St. Louis, Missouri
Chapter 4. Home Management of the Older Adult
  With Cancer

Enoch Albert, MS, RNC, OCN®
Patient Care Coordinator
Togus Veterans Administration Medical Center
Augusta, Maine
Chapter 11. Quality-of-Life Assessment for the Older
  Adult With Cancer

Sarah H. Dessner, MSN, RN, OCN®
Associate Professor of Nursing
Northern Kentucky University
Highland Heights, Kentucky
Chapter 2. Prevention and Detection

Barbara Duer, BSN, RN
Master's Degree Candidate
College of Nursing
University of Oklahoma
Oklahoma City, Oklahoma
Chapter 3. Interdisciplinary Management of the Older
  Adult With Cancer

Rhonda Kinsey, MSN, RN, AOCN®
Oncology Advanced Practice Nurse
Regional West Medical Center
Scottsbluff, Nebraska
Chapter 8. Treatment and Care of the Older Adult
  With Prostate Cancer

Terri Maxwell, RN, MSN, AOCN®
Executive Director

Palliative Care Center
Department of Family Medicine
Thomas Jefferson University
Philadelphia, Pennsylvania
Chapter 10. Symptom Management in the Older Adult
  With Cancer

Jacquelynn Nelson, RN, MSN, NP, C, AOCN®
Bellevue Hematology/Oncology, PC
Trenton, New Jersey
Chapter 10. Symptom Management in the Older Adult
  With Cancer

Beverly S. Reigle, PhD, RN
Assistant Professor
Department of Nursing
College of Mount St. Joseph
Cincinnati, Ohio
Chapter 6. Breast Cancer in Elderly Women

Alice G. Rini, JD, MS, RN
Associate Professor of Nursing and Law
Northern Kentucky University
Highland Heights, Kentucky
Chapter 13. Legal Issues in Cancer Nursing of the
  Older Adult

Judith Schneider, MSN, RN, CRNH
Manager, Hospice
Oncology Unit
St. Elizabeth Hospitals
Covington, Kentucky
Chapter 7. Treatment and Care of the Older Adult
  With Colorectal Cancer

Sandra Skorupa, RN, MS
Director of Nursing, Medical-Surgical/Critical Care
United Health Services Hospitals
Binghamton, New York
Chapter 12. Spiritual Care of the Older Adult With
  Cancer

Shirley S. Travis, PhD, RN, CS
Dean W. Colvard Distinguished Professor of Nursing
College of Nursing and Health Professions
University of North Carolina at Charlotte
Charlotte, North Carolina
Chapter 3. Interdisciplinary Management of the Older
  Adult With Cancer

Table of Contents

Foreword

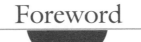

Betty Rolling Ferrell, PhD, RN, FAAN

In the late 1980s, I received an invitation as a "geriatric nurse" to write a paper for a geriatric journal. I was surprised by the invitation, and I explained to the editor that I was not a geriatric nurse; I was an oncology nurse! I went on to explain that I was a homecare nurse, a hospice nurse, a pain nurse, and a nurse researcher, but not a geriatric/gerontologic nurse! One of my colleagues, with some amusement, pointed out that although I did not think of myself as a gerontologic nurse, well over 80% of the patients in my studies were, in fact, elderly. Gerontologic nursing was not the field I had chosen, but it clearly was the work I was doing. This likely was my first step into the world of gerontologic oncology.

As we enter oncology care in the 21st century, most oncology nurses, with perhaps the exception of those focused exclusively on pediatrics, likely will realize that they are gerontologic nurses. But one does not just "become" a gerontologic oncology nurse by caring for the elderly any more than we "became" oncology nurses by virtue of caring for people with cancer. Becoming an oncology nurse has meant a very steep learning curve as we have acquired vast knowledge of cancer pathophysiology, chemotherapy, radiation therapy, and the supportive-care needs of people with cancer. The profession of gerontologic nursing also is based on a foundation of special knowledge in the care of older adults. To "become" gerontologic oncology nurses also will require intensive learning.

Handbook for the Care of the Older Adult With Cancer is designed to serve as a handbook to direct care. The content has been organized to draw us into the nursing world of gerontologic oncology through introductory chapters that describe demographic characteristics of older adults with cancer and the prevalence and detection of cancer in this population. The aging of our population and prevalence statistics remind us that gerontologic nursing is not some distant subspecialty but is, in fact, the work of virtually all oncology nurses. The chapter on interdisciplinary management of older adults addresses those issues that involve comprehensive patient care that cannot be given in isolation. It is through interdisciplinary collaboration that our older patients receive the care they so deserve.

The chapter on home management of patients with cancer is timely in an era of health system change and managed care. Just as virtually all oncology nurses are gerontologic oncology nurses, with certainty we know that virtually all patient care occurs in outpatient settings and the hospital room is now transposed to the living room.

I am reminded of the revolutionary changes that have occurred over my own career as an oncology nurse. I entered the profession in 1977 at a time prior to diagnosis-related groups (much less prior to managed care) when the solution to any concern related to care of an older patient was longer hospitalization. In less than 20 years, cancer care has evolved to outpatient treatment, wherein elderly spouses become homecare nurses and homes become treatment centers.

Handbook for the Care of the Older Adult With Cancer continues with a review of treatment of cancers that occur most commonly in older adults. The chapters in this section review these diseases, including lung, breast, colorectal, and prostate cancers. The content exemplifies the distinct nature of gerontologic nursing care. For example, although the pathophysiology of the disease of breast cancer may be very similar in young or middle-age women as compared to older women, the care of the 85-year-old woman with breast cancer is very unique. Care of older adults—the people with the cancer, not the tumor in the person—is strongly influenced by all aspects of aging, including physiologic processes of aging, psychological issues in the elderly, the social demand of aging, altered symptom response, and existential issues associated with encountering a life-threatening disease while also confronting the final phase of life.

The remaining chapters of *Handbook for the Care of the Older Adult With Cancer* move us further into the nursing world of gerontologic oncology. The chapters on cancer pain and symptom management remind us of the difficult tightrope we walk as oncology nurses. We balance on this tightrope the need to aggressively relieve pain and other symptoms that intensify suffering and destroy quality of life while preserving function and avoiding problems such as oversedation or medication interactions common in a population replete with concurrent illnesses.

While this book draws us into the world of gerontologic oncology, the chapter on quality of life in older adults with cancer is the universe encompassing it. Oncology nurses care for all aspects of living with cancer, including physical, psychological, social, and spiritual well-being. The chapter on spiritual care is not just a guide for referral to chaplaincy services but rather a guide for the spiritual assessment and intervention that is the responsibility of every nurse.

Entering the nursing world of gerontologic oncology is an essential component of providing cancer care in the new millennium. The complex demands of care for older adults with cancer challenge us but also enrich our lives, both personally and professionally. Let this book be your travel guide.

Preface

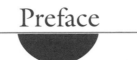

Nurses manage the care of older adult patients before, during, and after a cancer diagnosis and treatment. Nurses are concerned with the physical, emotional, and psychosocial outcomes of diagnosis and treatment as perceived by their patients. This book has been developed to aid nurses in the care of their older adult patients with cancer and in the prevention and early diagnosis of cancer.

The diagnosis of cancer most often is associated with the final stage of life. Family members and significant others frequently are ill-prepared to understand and manage the needs of older adults with cancer without assistance from nurses and other members of the healthcare team. Nurses usually are the primary healthcare professionals that provide anticipated needs with compassionate care to patients and families throughout this physically and emotionally charged ordeal. A nursing resource focused on the special needs of those caring for older adults with cancer is needed.

Nurses provide care to elderly patients with cancer in multiple settings, such as in offices and clinics, in homes, in hospitals, in hospices, and in long-term care facilities. The spectrum of care is broad, and nurses in each care setting should have in their repertoire knowledge of care needs across the healthcare spectrum. It also supports the communication between nurses in different settings, thus increasing the quality of care to their patients.

Physical and psychological care components are essential to the well-being of the care unit. This book expands that information to encompass quality-of-life issues and spiritual care. Legal issues also are included to address such matters as standards of nursing practice and bioethical end-of-life decisions that nurses often face.

The contributors to this book all have expertise in gerontology and oncology nursing. This coupling of two areas of expertise is a reasonable and logical one (albeit a rare one), as the major cancers occur with increasing frequency in older adults. Many nurses who care for older adults with cancer have little knowledge of the specialty of gerontologic nursing, which focuses on the special needs of older adults. Likewise, many nurses in general medical-surgical nursing and long-term care have minimal expertise with and knowledge of the special needs of patients with cancer. This book attempts to provide this knowledge.

Advanced practice nurses will benefit from the information in this handbook. They will gain knowledge that may not be found in their basic nurse practitioner or clinical nurse specialist nursing programs with a focus in adult, gerontology, or oncology nursing.

The size of this book was selected so as not to overwhelm the reader who wants immediate information for a pressing problem. It can be readily carried from office to patient location or other settings. It is meant to be easily used. The chapters are based on the specific needs of clinicians caring for these patients. It is further subdivided into relevant areas, again, to make it more useful to the healthcare providers.

The editors and contributors are very proud to have provided an opportunity for nurses from different specialties in gerontology and oncology to collaborate. We believe that all will benefit from that, including our respective organizations, the National Gerontological Nursing Association and Oncology Nursing Society. This is the first collaborative effort of members of these two groups.

Ann Schmidt Luggen, PhD, RN, CS, CNAA, ARNP
Sue E. Meiner, EdD, RN, CS, GNP

Chapter One

Demographic Data:
Cancer in Older Adults

Ann Schmidt Luggen, PhD, RN, CS, CNAA, ARNP

The lifespan of human beings has increased over the past 200 years. The number of older adults is growing, especially the oldest older adults. In these older age groups, cancer is a major cause of morbidity and mortality. Indeed, it is the second leading cause of death after heart disease.

One out of every two men is diagnosed with cancer in his lifetime; lung and prostate cancers are the most common (Cunningham, 1997). One in every three women is diagnosed with cancer in her lifetime (Parker, Tong, Bolden, & Wingo, 1997), predominately lung and breast cancers. Furthermore, cancer mortality is decreasing (American Cancer Society [ACS], 1998; McDonald, 1999); therefore, more older adults are living with cancer.

Cancer Data in Older Adults

The major invasive cancers in older adults, ages 60–79, are prostate, breast, lung and bronchus, and colon and rectal cancers. Data from the National Cancer Institute are shown in Table 1.1.

Leading Cancer Sites, American Men

Prostate Cancer

Prostate cancer is the most prevalent cancer in elderly men, followed by lung and bronchus, and colon and rectum. Prostate cancer accounts for 43% of new cancer cases (Parker et al., 1997). Between 1990 and 1997, prostate cancer incidence increased dramatically. Men aged 60–79 faced a one in six chance (17%) of developing prostate cancer. The lifetime risk was one in five, or nearly 20% (Parker et al.).

Today, men are being diagnosed with prostate cancer earlier. In 1986, only 38% of men were diagnosed before the age of 70, compared to 50% in 1993 (Menck, Jessup, &

Table 1.1 Percent of Older American Adults Developing Cancer, by Age

Cancer Type	40–59	60–79	Ever (birth to death)
Lung and bronchus			
Male	1.34 (1:75)	6.55 (1:15)	8.27 (1:12)
Female	0.97 (1:103)	3.95 (1:25)	5.64 (1:18)
Breast			
Female	4.00 (1:25)	6.88 (1:15)	5.69 (1:18)
Colorectal			
Male	0.87 (1:15)	4.05 (1:25)	5.69 (1:18)
Female	0.67 (1:50)	3.14 (1:32)	5.62 (1:18)
Prostate			
Male	1.83 (1:55)	14.79 (1:7)	17.00 (1:6)

Note. Based on information from Landis, Murray, Bolden, & Wingo, 1999.

Eyre, 1997). However, the proportion of stage II prostate cancer at diagnosis increased from 19% in 1986 to 48% in 1993 and the proportions of stages 0–I and IV declined (Menck et al.).

Treatment for prostate cancer has changed. Prostatectomy increased from 10% in 1986 to 29% in 1993. The proportion of patients receiving no therapy for prostate cancer declined from 43% in 1986 to 22% in 1993 (Menck et al., 1997).

Lung and Bronchus

The second most common invasive cancer in older men is lung and bronchus; 6.8% of men ages 60–79 will develop cancer in this site (Landis, Murray, Bolden, & Wingo, 1999). One in 15 men is at risk in this age group, and 1 in 12, or 8.6%, will be diagnosed with it in his lifetime. In an outcomes study of 12,000 patients with primary lung cancer, patterns of failure and relapse were similar in different histologic types of lung and bronchus cancer (Menck et al., 1997).

Colon and Rectum

Colorectal cancer is the third most common cancer in older men. Colorectal cancer occurs in 4.3% of men ages 60–79; 1 in 17 will be diagnosed with it in his lifetime (Landis et al., 1999). Colorectal cancer presents with earlier-stage disease in older adults (over 80) than in younger adults (Menck et al., 1997).

Leading Cancer Sites, American Women

Breast

Breast cancer is the most prevalent invasive cancer in women ages 60–79 (Landis et al., 1999). One in 14 older women will develop breast cancer, and 1 in 8 women will develop it in her lifetime. Breast cancer incidence increases with age up to 75–79 (481 cases in 100,000 women), but it then declines in women over 85 years old (451 cases in 100,000 women) (Leitch, Dodd, & Costanza, 1997).

Breast cancer is known to grow faster in young women compared to elderly women (Leitch et al., 1997), and older women have less-aggressive breast cancer compared to younger women (Menck et al., 1997). ACS recommends annual mammography for women beginning at age 40 to aid in the screening process and early diagnosis (Leitch et al.). The organization does not specify an age at which screening should be terminated. However, National Cancer Data Bank (NCDB) data analysis of women 75 and older found fewer cancers diagnosed in this age group with mammography. Also, needle biopsy is performed less often in this age group (Menck et al.).

Lung and Bronchus; Colon and Rectum

The second most prevalent cancer in older women is lung and bronchus, followed by colon and rectum. Women who are 60–79 years old have a 1 in 26 chance of developing lung cancer but a lifetime risk of 1 in 18 (Landis et al., 1999) (see Table 1.1). Colorectal cancer occurs in about 3% of women ages 60–79 and 5.8% of women from birth to death. All three cancers increase with aging.

Cancer Deaths in Older Adults

The number of deaths from cancer continues to increase because of the aging U.S. population (Parker et al., 1997). Although preliminary data from 1995 suggest that mortality rates are declining, in fact, the number of deaths is increasing (ACS, 1998). An estimated 563,100 Americans died with cancer in 1998, more than 1,500 people each day (McDonald, 1999).

Deaths from all cancer sites are the same in men and women over age 75 but are higher in men ages 55–74 (142,057 in men compared to 111,937 in women of the same age).

Cancer deaths in men are predominantly caused by lung and bronchus cancer in both the 55–74 and 75+ age groups (see Table 1.2) (Parker et al., 1997). Colorectal cancer is the second leading cause of cancer death in the United States. Six percent of Americans will develop it in their lifetime (Byers, Levin, Rothenberger, Dodd, & Smith, 1997). Early detection can prevent morbidity and mortality. Colorectal cancer deaths are higher in the younger elderly group (55–74), but prostate cancer is higher in the older elderly group (75+).

Since 1987, lung and bronchus cancers have been responsible for the greatest number of cancer deaths in older women (Parker et al., 1997). Prior to that, breast cancer caused more deaths and was the leading cause of cancer death for 40 years. In 1995, breast cancer was the cause of 17% of deaths (Parker et al.), killing nearly 20,000 women per year in the 60–79-year-old group and nearly 10,000 per year in the 80+ group (Landis et al., 1999). Colorectal cancer kills more elderly women (80+) than breast cancer; it is the third leading cause of cancer death in older women ages 60–79 (Landis et al.).

Table 1.2. Leading Cancer Sites, Reported Deaths by Age and Sex—1993

Cancer Site	Cases in Males		Cases in Females	
	Age 55–74	Age 75+	Age 55–74	Age 75+
Lung	55,421	28,122	31,803	18,802
Colorectal	13,689	11,787	10,861	16,137
Prostate	12,051	22,465	—	—
Breast	—	—	18,937	14,778

Note. Based on information from Parker, Tong, Bolden, & Wingo, 1997.

Racial and Ethnic Variables in Cancer Incidence and Deaths

Caucasians are the largest racial group in the United States, representing about 84% of the population, according to 1990 U.S. census data (ACS, 1997). Hispanics comprised about 9% of the population in the 1990 census, but their numbers are expected to rise to 23% of the population by 2050. Black Americans numbered about 30 million (12%) in the last census. Asian and Pacific Islanders represented 3%, but their numbers are expected to increase to nearly 11% by 2050. Native Americans, including American Indians and Alaskan Natives, represented about 0.8% of the U.S. population. Cancer data on American Indians is available only from New Mexico (ACS, 1997).

Cancer in Older Adults: Data for Black and White Americans

Breast cancer occurs more commonly in white women than black women, but more black women are diagnosed at later stages than white women (Landis et al., 1999). Prostate cancer occurs more in black men than white men (180.6/100,000 and 134.7/100,000 respectively) (ACS, 1998). Regional spread at diagnosis also is more common in white Americans, but elderly black men are diagnosed more often with distant metastases than elderly white men and are more likely to die with prostate cancer (McDonald, 1999).

Lung and bronchus cancers are similar in both white and black groups in terms of localized, regional, and distant spread at diagnosis. However, blacks experience a slight increase in the incidence of distant metastases at diagnosis—44% compared to 49% in whites (Parker et al., 1997).

Colorectal cancer data are similar in both groups. Localized cancer represents 38% of cancers in whites and 32% of cancers in blacks. Regional spread at diagnosis is 37% in whites and 36% in blacks. Distant metastases at diagnosis is 19% in whites and 25% in blacks (Parker et al., 1997).

Black and White Survival Rates After Cancer Diagnosis

White women have higher five-year survival rates compared to black women at all stages of diagnosis of breast cancer (85% compared to 70%) (see Table 1.3.).

Prostate cancer five-year survival is greater in white males (89%) compared to blacks (73%) (Parker et al., 1997). For localized prostate cancer, the five-year survival is 100% in whites and 91% in blacks. For regional spread, the survival rate is 94% in whites and 80% in blacks. With distant metastases, the survival rate is 31% for whites and 25% for blacks (Parker et al.).

The lung cancer scenario is similar to that of other cancers, with an increased five-year survival for whites compared to blacks. The difference is not as disparate as prostate cancer, though. Five-year survival at all stages is 14% for whites and 11% for blacks (see Table 1.4).

The colorectal cancer five-year survival is, for all stages, 62% in whites and 53% in blacks (Parker et al., 1997) (see Table 1.5).

Racial and Ethnic Data on Cancer in Older Adults

ACS estimated that 531,000 cancer deaths occurred in the United States in 1999 (Landis et al., 1999). Of these deaths, 483,500 were in white Americans, 62,200 were in black Americans, and 14,300 were among other racial and ethnic U.S. groups (ACS, 1997). In men, cancer inci-

Table 1.3. Black and White Women Five-Year Survival Rates for Breast Cancer

Cancer Type	White Women	Black Women
Localized	97%	89%
Regional	77%	61%
Distant metastases	21%	16%

Note. Based on information from Parker, Tong, Bolden, & Wingo, 1997.

Table 1.4. Black and White Women Five-Year Survival Rates for Lung Cancer

Cancer Type	White Women	Black Women
Localized	49%	43%
Regional	18%	14%
Distant metastases	2%	2%

Note. Based on information from Parker, Tong, Bolden, & Wingo, 1997.

Table 1.5. Black and White Women Five-Year Survival Rates for Colorectal Cancer

Cancer Type	White Women	Black Women
Localized	92%	86%
Regional	64%	60%
Distant metastases	7%	5%

Note. Based on information from Parker, Tong, Bolden, & Wingo, 1997.

dence is highest in blacks, followed by whites (16% less). Cancer incidence is lowest in American Indians in New Mexico, although it is also low in Asian Americans of Chinese, Korean, and Filipino descent. The cancer mortality rate for African Americans is 224.8 per 100,000, which is higher than for any other ethnic or racial group (McDonald, 1999).

In women, rates across racial and ethnic groups are similar. Cancer rates are highest in Alaskan native women, with U.S. white women next. Cancer is lowest in American Indian women from New Mexico and Korean Americans but is also low in Chinese and Filipino women (ACS, 1997).

Black Americans: Black Americans comprise 12% of the U.S. population according to the 1990 census (ACS, 1997). Sites of cancer with the highest incidence in black males are prostate, lung, colorectal, oral, and stomach. Black males have the highest overall incidence of cancer compared to any other racial or ethnic group in the United States.

Rates of cancer in black women are higher than in any racial or ethnic group except Alaskan Native women (ACS, 1997). The leading cancer sites in black women are lung, breast, colorectal, uterus, and cervix (Landis et al., 1999).

A major risk factor for U.S. blacks seems to be obesity. According to data reported by ACS (1997), nearly 38% of black women and 28% of black men are overweight. Black women are more likely to be overweight compared to all other races and ethnic groups.

Native Americans: Native Americans include American Indians and Alaskan Natives. They comprise less than 1% of the U.S. population (ACS, 1997). Cancers with the highest incidence in American Indian men are prostate, lung and bronchus, and colorectal (Landis et al.,

1999). The incidence of kidney cancer is higher in American Indians than in any other group (ACS, 1997).

American Indian women have a high incidence of breast, ovarian, colorectal, and gallbladder cancers. Overall, cancer rates are lower in American Indians than other racial or ethnic groups. How representative these data are, however, is unclear (ACS, 1997).

Alaskan Native men have a high incidence of lung, colorectal, and prostate cancer; colorectal cancer prevalence is higher in Alaskan Natives than in any other racial or ethnic group (ACS, 1997). Alaskan Native women experience a high incidence of breast, colorectal, and lung cancer. These women have the highest rates of colorectal and lung cancer of any race or ethnic group.

Asian/Pacific Islanders: This group comprises about 3% of the U.S. population according to the 1990 census (ACS, 1997). Included in Asian/Pacific Islanders are people of Chinese, Filipino, Hawaiian, Japanese, Korean, and Vietnamese heritage.

The cancers with the highest incidence in Chinese, Filipino, Hawaiian, and Japanese American men are prostate, lung, and colorectal. Among Korean American men, cancers with the highest incidence include lung, stomach, and colorectal; among Vietnamese American men, cancers with high incidence are lung, liver, and prostate. Rates of stomach cancer in Korean American men and liver cancer in Vietnamese American men are higher than in any other racial or ethnic group (ACS, 1997).

Among Asian/Pacific Islander women, breast, colorectal, and lung and bronchus cancers are highest in incidence (Landis et al., 1999). Stomach cancer is the leading cancer in American women of Japanese and Korean heritage (ACS, 1997). The rate of cervical cancer is highest in Vietnamese American women; cervical cancer rates are more than two and a half times higher in this group than in any other racial or ethnic group.

Whites: Caucasians comprise 84% of the U.S. population (ACS, 1997). In white men, prostate, lung, colorectal, bladder, and non-Hodgkin's lymphoma are cancers with the highest incidence rates. White men have the highest incidence of bladder cancer compared to any racial or ethnic group—two times higher than Hispanic men, who have the second highest incidence.

Breast, lung, colorectal, uterine, and ovarian cancer are the cancers with the highest incidence in white women (ACS, 1997). The incidence of breast cancer in white women is higher than in any racial or ethnic group (Landis et al., 1999).

Hispanics: This group represents 9% of the U.S. population (ACS, 1997). The most common cancer sites in Hispanic Americans are the same as those in white Americans, but the incidence rates are about 30% lower. The rate of cervical cancer is very high in Hispanic American women.

Geographic Data

Five U.S. states report the highest incidence of new cancer cases that affect elderly Americans. These states are California, New York, Florida, Texas, and Pennsylvania. The estimated new cases for 1999 are listed in Table 1.6 (Landis et al., 1999).

Cancer mortality data by the state are very similar to new case data. The same five states have the highest number of cancer deaths of older adults in the United States.

Cancer in Long-Term Care Settings

Data regarding cancer in older adults who live in long-term care settings are not easily obtained. In 1981, the National Nursing Home Survey reported that 2.7% of residents had cancer as a first or second diagnosis (U.S. Department of Health and Human Services, 1981).

Table 1.6. Estimated New Cancer Cases Affecting Older Adult Americans—1997

Geographic Area	Prostate Cancer	Lung Cancer	Breast Cancer	Colorectal Cancer
California	16,300	14,600	16,900	11,200
Florida	13,600	13,000	11,900	8,900
Texas	11,600	11,500	11,300	11,300
New York	11,500	10,700	13,000	9,400
Pennsylvania	9,900	9,000	10,000	7,700
United States	179,000	171,000	175,000	129,000

Note. Based on information from Landis, Murray, Bolden, & Wingo, 1999.

Conclusion

Cancer is a major health concern in the U.S. and in the world. Most cancers occur in older adults. It appears that some cancers are decreasing in incidence. Prostate cancer has declined 28% between 1992 and 1995 (after increasing 85% between 1987 and 1992) (Landis et al., 1999). For all sites, cancer incidence has declined 0.7% per year from 1990 and 1995, contrasting with increasing incidence in earlier years. However, it should be known that the U.S. doesn't have a national cancer registry. Therefore, all cancer cases are estimates made from the U.S. Bureau of Census data (Landis et al.).

The rate of cancer deaths appears to be leveling and even declining. The incidence of lung and bronchus cancers has decreased in men 2.3% per year between 1990 and 1995. The incidence of lung cancer in women has stabilized. However, the number of breast cancer cases has been increasing since 1988 (Landis et al., 1999).

There is an urgent need to address the special concerns of older adults. The need for prevention and control strategies and cancer treatment and care is great and is likely to increase (Freeman, 1997). Oncology nurses and gerontology nurses have an obligation to learn as much as they can about the care of this special population of older adults who bear the burden of these diseases—cancer. This book is one effort to assist in this endeavor.

References

American Cancer Society. (1997). *Cancer facts & figures—1997*. Atlanta: Author.

American Cancer Society. (1998). *Cancer facts & figures—1998*. Atlanta: Author.

Byers, T., Levin, B., Rothenberger, D., Dodd, G.D., & Smith, R.A. (1997). ACS guidelines for screening and surveillance for early detection of colorectal polyps and cancer: Update 1997. *CA: A Cancer Journal for Clinicians, 47*, 154–160.

Cunningham, M.P. (1997). Cancer, giving life to numbers. *CA: A Cancer Journal for Clinicians, 47*, 3–4.

Freeman, H. (1997, July 17). *President's Cancer Panel. Cancer and the aging population* [Online]. Available: http://deainfo.nci.nih.gov/advisory/pcp/pcp0797/minutes.html [1999, March 18].

Landis, S., Murray, T., Bolden, S., & Wingo, P.A. (1999). Cancer statistics: 1999. *CA: A Cancer Journal for Clinicians, 49*, 8–31.

Leitch, A.M., Dodd, G.D., & Costanza, M. (1997). American Cancer Society guidelines for the early detection of breast cancer: Update 1997. *CA: A Cancer Journal for Clinicians, 47*, 150–153.

McDonald, C.J. (1999). Cancer statistics, 1999: Challenges in minority populations. *CA: A Cancer Journal for Clinicians, 49,* 6–7.

Menck, H.R., Jessup, J.M., & Eyre, H.J. (1997). Clinical highlights from the National Cancer Data Base: 1997. *CA: A Cancer Journal for Clinicians, 47,* 161–170.

Parker, S.L., Tong, T., Bolden, S., & Wingo, P.A. (1997). Cancer statistics, 1997. *CA: A Cancer Journal for Clinicians, 47,* 5–27.

U.S. Department of Health and Human Services. (1981). *Characteristics of nursing home residents, health status and care received: National nursing home survey* [DHHS Public Health Service Publication # 81-1712]. Rockville, MD: Author.

Chapter Two

Prevention and Detection

Sarah H. Dessner, MSN, OCN®

Introduction

A discussion of cancer prevention in the elderly must begin with the understanding that the most significant risk factor for the major cancers in this population is increasing age (Fitch et al., 1997). Cancer incidence of all sites significantly increases with advancing age, as more than half of all cancers diagnosed annually in the United States occur in individuals over 65 years of age and 60% of cancer deaths occur in older people (Goldberg & Chavin, 1997). Advanced age also is associated with a more advanced stage of cancer at the initial diagnosis. Although effective treatments and survival rates have improved over the past 40 years, the cancer death rate among older adults remains high (Robinson & Beghe, 1997). A concern for practitioners caring for older adults is that, traditionally, this population has not been targeted for prevention, screening, and early detection (Boyle, 1996). Many practitioners hold the belief that early detection efforts are not appropriate for this population because aggressive medical intervention should not be pursued in older adults with cancer (Fitch et al.). Others identify the benefit of early detection of cancer in older adults as a way to limit or reduce morbidity and suffering (Blesch & Prohaska, 1991; Mandelblatt et al., 1992; Robinson & Beghe). Goals for prevention, risk reduction, and early detection in older people not only should target decreasing morbidity and mortality but also should include the preservation of function and quality of life (Goldberg & Chavin, 1997). Traditionally, the primary focus of medical and nursing science has been on the treatment of cancer. Only recently have health promotion and disease prevention been emphasized (List, 1992). The concept of eliminating or modifying neoplastic transformation of human cells has become a goal for prevention and detection programs.

As a nonmodifiable risk factor, longevity must be accepted as a constant as the healthcare community considers ways to decrease the overall risk to older clients for developing cancer. Recent data suggest that overall cancer mortality rates are beginning to decline. The numbers of deaths, however, continue to climb because of a rapidly increasing aging population. Although estimates of new cancer cases and cancer deaths vary considerably from year to year, these estimates provide an indication of the patterns of cancer incidence in the United States. Clearly, continued prevention and screening efforts are needed to address the increasing cancer incidence because the older adult population will continue to rise dramatically into the 21st century (Parker, Tong, Bolden, & Wingo, 1997). At the beginning of the 20th century, the average 65-year-old woman was expected to live 12 more years. The same woman would be expected to live 20 or more years if she were 65 today (Rubenstein & Nahas, 1998).

In 1992, the Oncology Nursing Society (ONS) recognized the special needs of older adults in a position paper mandating that oncology nursing address the special needs of older patients with cancer. Included in the statement, which outlines the areas to be addressed, is cancer prevention and early detection activities for older adults (Boyle et al., 1992). More than half of all patients with cancer are, or soon will be, over 65 years of age. Therefore, this population must be aggressively included in programs to stimulate compliance with risk minimization and early detection. In this era of cost consciousness in health care, much of the emphasis on preventative measures and slowing functional decline may be driven by economics (Ebersole, 1998). In addition, ONS (1998) issued the Patients' Bill of Rights for Quality Cancer Care. This document supports access to education about cancer prevention and availability of screening activities for early detection of cancer as rights for all individuals.

Prevention of Cancer in Older Adults

Practitioners involved in the prevention of cancer in older adults must address ways to affect successful prevention programs for individuals throughout their lives. For many types of cancer, lifestyle habits and possible exposure to carcinogens result in a cumulative effect over an individual's lifetime. If the goal is to prevent cancer in older adults, preventative practices must start early in life (Goldberg & Chavin, 1997). A healthy lifestyle and good medical care throughout an individual's lifetime may prevent or delay some risk factors for cancer (primary prevention) and eliminate or minimize some preexisting conditions (secondary prevention). Healthy lifestyle and good medical care ultimately may minimize morbidity and loss of quality of life caused by established malignant disease (tertiary prevention) (Goldberg & Chavin).

Many factors related to carcinogenesis may play a role in the development of cancer with increasing age. Causal factors act together or in sequence to initiate or promote carcinogenesis. Often, 10 or more years may pass between the time the individual is exposed to a carcinogen and when mutation or detectable cancer occurs (American Cancer Society [ACS], 1998). Theories related to the predominance of cancer in older adults (Boyle, 1994; Cohen, 1994) include
- Length of carcinogen exposure
- Accumulation of somatic mutations
- Decreased ability to repair DNA
- Oncogene activation or amplification
- Tumor suppressor gene loss
- Decreased immune surveillance
- Increased sensitivity to oncogenic viruses
- Increased tendency for hormone imbalance.

Guidelines for Prevention

In offering counseling and education to older adults, healthcare providers must be aware of the challenge to change or improve lifestyle habits that may have existed for many years.

ACS publishes guidelines that advise the public about practices that research has shown to reduce the risks of developing malignant disease. Expert advisory committees develop the guidelines, which are based on the most recent available scientific evidence using studies in human populations and laboratory research.

Overview of Guidelines for Prevention

The evidence reflected in these guidelines suggests that as many as one-third of the cancer deaths that occurred in the United States during 1998 were the result of dietary factors. Approximately 175,000 cancer deaths were related to tobacco use, and an additional 19,000 cancer deaths were related to excessive alcohol use, frequently in combination with tobacco use (ACS, 1998; Parker et al., 1997). The combined use of tobacco and alcohol has a cancer-causing effect that is greater than the use of either product alone (Cheng & Day; 1996, Marshall & Boyle, 1996). The most significant modifiable risk factors are poor dietary choices, smoking, alcohol use, and physical inactivity (ACS 1996 Advisory Committee on Diet Nutrition and Cancer Prevention, 1996). Changes in health habits, which include smoking cessation, improved dietary practices with limited alcohol use, and increased regular physical activity, may be beneficial in decreasing an older adult's risk of developing cancer. In addition to the protective effect of specific food groups, the overall improved health that results from a healthy diet and physical activity increases the immune system's ability to protect against cancer and other diseases. In general, these guidelines for older adults are recommended for individuals of all ages.

Nutritional Guidelines for Cancer Prevention

Fruits and vegetables: High consumption of fruits and vegetables has been shown to protect against many cancers, including colon, breast, and lung. The positive effect of increased fruits and vegetables in the diet has even been demonstrated in individuals who smoke. Studies show that smokers' diets tend to be less nutritious than nonsmokers' diets. These individuals still may benefit from a diet high in fruits and vegetables. Lung cancer risk in both smokers and nonsmokers has been shown to decrease in individuals who consume large amounts of vegetables and fruits (Zeigler, Mayne, & Swanson, 1996).

Fruits and vegetables are rich sources of many beneficial anticancer compounds including vitamin C, carotenes, flavonoids, and trace minerals. These compounds are known as antioxidants because they protect against damage produced by highly reactive molecules that bind to and destroy cellular components. The highly reactive molecules are called free radicals and are thought to play a role in aging as well as in the development of cancer and other diseases. The most important of the antioxidant nutrients are thought to be vitamin C and the carotenes. The best sources of carotenes are dark-green, leafy vegetables, such as kale, collard greens, mustard greens, and spinach, and yellow and orange fruits and vegetables, such as apricots, cantaloupe, carrots, sweet potatoes, yams, and squash. Red and purple vegetables and fruits, such as berries, plums, tomatoes, and red cabbage, also are good sources.

Another family of vegetables that ACS recommends for its ability to reduce cancer risk is the cabbage family. These vegetables also are known as cruciferous vegetables and include cabbage, broccoli, cauliflower, brussels sprouts, rutabagas, turnips, radishes, and other common vegetables.

Grains: The addition of fiber-rich foods, such as whole-grain breads, cereals, and grain products, including rice, pasta, and beans, is associated with a decreased risk for gastrointestinal cancers. These foods decrease bowel transit time for the colon contents. The effect is a decrease in the concentration of absorbable bowel toxins and metabolites. In addition, these foods provide many nutrients other than fiber that add to overall health. Legumes, soybeans, and foods produced from soybeans, grains, and seeds contain cancer-fighting carotenes. Another food source thought to play a role in cancer prevention is garlic and foods prepared with garlic (Dausch & Nixon, 1990; Messina & Barnes, 1991).

Animal fats: A diet high in animal fats has been associated with an increased risk for cancers of the gastrointestinal tract, prostate, and endometrium. A diet that limits animal fat intake is recommended for cancer prevention. In the older adult population, an important side benefit to a low-fat diet is the potential for decreasing the risk for coronary artery disease and cerebral vascular accident.

Factors Affecting Diet in Older Adults

Compliance with eating a healthy diet, rich in cancer-fighting foods, may be difficult for older adults. Problems that may affect dietary practices include a decreased appetite and loss of interest in eating. Normal aging results in a decrease in saliva and atrophy of the taste buds. Aging also may result in changes in the ability to chew and digest foods. Older adults commonly face emotional issues, such as depression and grief, which negatively affect appetite. Certain illnesses prevalent in older adults, such as dementia, result in changes in appetite and the inability to follow guidelines for good nutrition. Financial restraints and access to markets often impact the availability of some foods for older adults. Healthcare providers must be creative in developing ways to ensure that their older patients receive healthy and varied diets that are palatable and prepared for their specific needs (Andresen, 1998).

Physical Activity Programs for Older Adults

Physical activity and avoiding obesity have been shown to reduce the risk of cancer through several mechanisms. For breast and prostate cancer, the effect may be related to the production of hormones. Obesity has been linked to an increase in estrogen levels in postmenopausal women (Hill & Austin, 1996). Other cancers that may be caused in part by lack of activity or associated obesity include gastrointestinal cancer and prostate, endometrium, breast, and kidney cancers (ACS 1996 Advisory Committee on Diet, Nutrition, and Cancer Prevention, 1996). The relationship between increased physical activity and lower incidence of gastrointestinal cancer may be because of exercise's ability to reduce bowel transit time and an associated decrease in exposure of the colonic mucosa to bile acids (Strohl, 1998).

Increasing older adults' physical activity may present a considerable challenge for healthcare providers. Individuals who have been active throughout their lives are likely to continue that pattern as long as they are physically able. Those who have enjoyed more sedentary lifestyles or have never learned a sport or other physically active pastime may be resistant to the idea of beginning such activities late in life. In addition, underlying physical conditions that are common in older adults, such as arthritis and coronary artery disease, may prohibit initiation of physical activity.

Group exercise programs designed for older age groups and conducted with sensitivity to the participants' abilities may help to encourage activity. Older adults should be encouraged to wear comfortable, loose-fitting clothes with shoes that offer adequate support and comfort. Some individuals may have poor flexibility or a history of joint disease, resulting in an inability or difficulty to comfortably stand or lie on the floor. Providing a straight-backed chair for these individuals and modifying the exercises to accommodate disabilities may encourage participation. Any movement is good, but exercises should never cause pain.

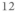

As with many activities, most older adults respond better to activities that they can do with others of their same age. If music is used during the exercise programs, consider participants' tastes in making selections. Individuals who live alone or prefer to exercise in private may benefit from carefully selected audiovisual exercise programs designed with the older adult in mind. Walking, swimming, and bicycle riding are all good activities for older adults and will be enjoyed more if performed with family, friends, or groups of individuals with similar interests and abilities.

Older adults should be reminded to avoid exposure to ultraviolet light to decrease the risk of skin cancer. Nurses should encourage use of sunscreens for individuals enjoying outdoor activities (Rubenstein & Nahas, 1998).

All individuals beginning a physical-activity program late in life should begin gradually. The healthcare provider should be consulted about any limitations or restrictions that must be considered in planning an individualized exercise program.

Tobacco and Alcohol Use in the Elderly

ACS estimated that in 1998, about 175,000 deaths resulted from tobacco use and an additional 19,000 cancer deaths were related to excessive alcohol, frequently in combination with tobacco use (Parker et al., 1997). Cancers caused by cigarette smoking and heavy alcohol use could be prevented completely with effective cessation programs. Alcohol, along with tobacco products that are smoked, is associated with cancers of the oral cavity, esophagus, and larynx. Studies also show a relationship between alcohol use and an increased incidence of breast cancer. The risk of cancer related to drinking is associated with the amount consumed and may begin to rise with as little as two alcoholic drinks per day. The combined use of alcohol and smoking results in an effect greater than the use of each substance alone (Parker et al.). Current guidelines for alcohol consumption suggest that individuals who already use alcohol should limit their intake to one drink per day for women and two drinks per day for men (U.S. Department of Agriculture & U.S. Department of Health and Human Services, 1995). The difference in the guideline for women and men is based on the fact that women have a smaller body size and are less able to tolerate alcohol. In addition, women, particularly those with a family history of breast cancer, need to be aware of alcohol as a risk factor for this disease.

Moderate alcohol use, described as two drinks per day, has been shown to decrease the risk of coronary artery disease in middle-aged adults. Therefore, the benefit in terms of heart disease may outweigh the risk of cancer in men over 50 and in women over 60 (Ashley & Ferrence, 1994).

Smoking-Cessation Guidelines

Smoking cessation must be strongly recommended to all clients. Health practitioners should provide smoking-cessation counseling and referral to accessible smoking cessation programs. Treatment with nicotine-replacement products should be considered as an adjunct to smoking-cessation programs. Counseling may need to be repeated many times to deliver multiple messages. Some individuals may have the misconception that long-term smoking effects are irreversible and, therefore, smoking cessation will not benefit them. Educating these individuals regarding the positive results of smoking cessation at any age is important (Goldberg & Chavin, 1997). Healthcare providers must send a strong message in educating clients against smoking (see Figure 2.1).

Figure 2.1. Guidelines to Assist Those Who Indicate a Willingness to Stop Smoking

- Advise all smokers to stop smoking.
- Be clear in the importance of smoking cessation. "As your healthcare provider, I must advise you to stop smoking now."
- Personalize the message by referring to the patient's clinical condition, family history, social roles, and obligations.
- Help the smoker establish a specific date to stop smoking. Consider establishing a contract with the individual.
- If another family member agrees to stop along with the older adult, he or she can provide additional support.
- Offer nicotine-replacement therapy if medically appropriate.
- Stress that total abstinence is important.
- Explain that alcohol use may lead to relapse of smoking.
- Provide follow-up to review progress.

Note. Based on information from Dickey, 1994.

Guidelines for a Healthy Lifestyle

Many pamphlets and patient-teaching materials dealing with cancer prevention and healthy lifestyle are available. They are designed for the lay public and are suitable for the older adult population. Some resources for materials include ACS, American Institute for Cancer Research, U.S. Department of Agriculture, U.S. Department of Health and Human Services, and National Institutes of Health. In addition, Berendt (1998) suggested the following guidelines for a healthy lifestyle.

1. Eat two to four servings of fruits each day.
2. Eat three to five servings of vegetables each day. (Cruciferous, dark-green, and deep-yellow and orange vegetables are preferred.)
3. Snack on fruits and vegetables.
4. Include some fruits and vegetables in each meal.
5. Eat 6–11 servings per day of foods from plant sources, such as breads, cereals, grains, rice, pasta, and beans.
6. Include grains with every meal. Whole grains are preferable to processed grains.
7. Beans provide a good alternative to meat.
8. Limit intake of high-fat foods. Instead, choose foods low in fat.
9. Limit fat to two to three servings per day
10. Limit consumption of meats, especially high-fat meats. Instead, eat skinless poultry, fish, and lean meats.
11. Include two to three servings per day of dairy products, such as milk, yogurt, and cheese.
12. Limit consumption of salt-cured, smoked, and nitrite-preserved foods.
13. Stay or become physically active and maintain a healthy weight.
14. Participate in physical activities at least three days every week for 30 minutes or more at a time.
15. Stay within the healthy weight range for age.
16. Limit consumption of alcoholic beverages.
17. Do not smoke.

Screening and Early Detection in Older Adults

The best method for decreasing cancer morbidity and mortality is through early detection of cancer and effective early treatment. Studies support the effectiveness of screening programs for older adults (Chen, Tabar, Fagerberg, & Duffy, 1995). When discussing screening for a population of older adults, nurses should inform patients that advancing age alone puts older adults at risk for many cancers. Research has shown that cancer in older adults tends to be diagnosed at more advanced stages than cancer in younger individuals (Goodwin et al., 1986). Older adults tend to seek health care for their symptoms when their cancer has reached more advanced stages (Ouslander & Beck, 1982).

Detection examinations, tests, and procedures used in cancer-screening programs are not usually diagnostic alone. Detection measures identify people who require follow-up diagnostic procedures to rule out cancer (National Cancer Institute [NCI], 1997). In older adults, the concept of secondary prevention becomes significant. Secondary prevention involves defining and identifying individuals, or groups of individuals, who have the potential to develop cancer before symptoms develop. The emphasis is on early diagnosis and prompt treatment. Secondary prevention employs the use of screening strategies to detect disease in patients who are asymptomatic when the disease may be localized. Treatment at this stage is more likely to be effective in decreasing morbidity and mortality (Morrison, Olsen, & Ashley, 1998).

In considering methods to improve compliance with early-detection programs, potential reasons that cancers are diagnosed later in older adults must be considered. Addressing these issues may significantly impact compliance with screening programs and early detection of cancer in this population.

One reason that older adults may report symptoms late or not at all is that they assume the symptoms they are experiencing are age-related. Another reason may be a lack of knowledge about the symptoms that are warning signs for cancer. In addition, individuals may believe the symptoms are related to other preexisting illnesses (Satariano, Belle, & Swanson, 1986).

Screening Guidelines

The screening practices and programs in this population must be well established and strictly followed. Guidelines for detection of cancer in older adults should follow ACS standards. Age 85 has been proposed as a point beyond which conventional screening practices may not show continued benefit. A plan to continue screening beyond age 85 should be individualized to the specific patient (Goldberg & Chavin, 1997).

Cancer-Related Annual Checkup

ACS recommends that all older adults undergo a thorough cancer-directed history and physical examination annually. Figure 2.2 provides the elements of the annual examination. The examination should include health counseling related to tobacco control, sun exposure, diet and nutrition, and risk factors, as well as specific screening tests based on ACS recommendations (ACS, 1998; Boyle et al., 1992).

Figure 2.2. Annual Screening Examination for All Older Adults

The examination should include
- Total skin review
- Cervix
- Oral cavity
- Pelvis
- Thyroid
- Testicles
- Lymph
- Rectum
- Breasts
- Prostate

History

A patient history should include questions to obtain information needed to establish a risk profile. Age, sex, race, place of birth and childhood, and occupation all should be considered related to possible risk factors. Past medical history, especially related to malignant disease, should be obtained as well as a detailed family cancer history. Occupational history is important in assessing older adults so that cumulative exposure to possible carcinogens can be determined. Place of birth and childhood are important for the same reason. A history of smoking, drinking, sexual habits, and drug use may point to cancer risks. Due to a lack of information, many healthcare professionals tend to overlook the possibility of these behaviors as risk factors in older adults.

Symptom Review

A symptom review should be directed toward identifying any possible symptoms of malignant disease. If any symptoms are reported, a complete analysis of the symptoms must be performed. Professionals engaged in a workup of symptoms in older adults must be suspicious of specific and nonspecific symptoms. Complaints such as weight loss, anorexia, malaise, and altered bowel habits should not be attributed automatically to nonmalignant causes (Boyle et al., 1992). Symptoms should be considered warning signs for cancer in older adults as they are in all patients (see Figure 2.3 and Table 2.1).

Ovarian Cancer Screening

In patients with a family history of ovarian cancer, consideration may be given to a screening transvaginal sonography and/or serum CA 125 in addition to the physical exam. Physical examination alone is often inadequate in detecting ovarian cancer (Teneriello & Park, 1995).

Figure 2.3. Cancer Symptom Review for Older Adults

- Unusual weight loss or gain
- Onset of weakness, fatigue, or malaise
- Changes in warts or moles
- Lymphadenopathy or lymph node tenderness
- Cough, pain, dyspnea, or hemoptysis
- Change in appetite, pain, nausea, vomiting, change in bowel habits, or change in diameter or shape of stools
- Change in urinary pattern, hematuria, change in force or caliber of stream, or dysuria
- Postmenopausal bleeding, discharge, enlarged abdominal girth, bloating
- Flushing, sweating, tachycardia, palpitations, polyuria, polydipsia, or appetite disturbance
- Brushing and petechiae, anemia, or purpura
- Headache, vertigo, seizures, visual disturbances, or sensory or cognitive deficits
- Fever, chills, or frequent infections

Table 2.1. Symptom Confusion and Age-Related Problems

Possible Malignancy	Symptom/Sign	Non-Cancer Cause
Melanoma, or squamous cell carcinoma	Increased skin pigmentation	"Age spots"
Colon or rectum	Rectal bleeding	Hemorrhoids
Rectal	Constipation	"Old age"
Lung	Dyspnea	Getting old or out of shape
Prostate	Decreased urinary stream	Benign "dribbling" Prostatic hypertrophy
Breast	Breast contour change	"Normal" atrophy or fibrosis
Metastatic or other	Fatigue	Energy loss from aging
	Bone pain	Arthritis; "aches and pains" of aging

Cervical Cancer Screening

The diagnosis of new cervical cancer is not common in older women. However, women over 65 years of age who have not had negative Pap smear results documented should be screened yearly for two years and then at the discretion of the provider (Rubenstein & Nahas, 1998). At the present time, Medicare will pay for Pap screening every two years (Goldberg & Chavin, 1997).

Breast Cancer Screening

Mammography screening studies for breast cancer show a lower mortality rate in women ages 50–64 who have received yearly mammograms. The benefit to women older than 65 years of age has not been shown because of the low recruitment of this age group into studies (Harrison et al., 1997). ACS and NCI recommend yearly mammograms for women over age 50 with no upper age limit. The American Geriatrics Society supports mammography in older women every two to three years until at least age 85. The Forum for Breast Cancer Screening in Older Women recommends clinical breast exam yearly for women over 75 whose health and life expectancy remain good. Individual decisions to continue screening should be based on the knowledge that early detection and treatment will delay mortality and suffering in women of all age groups. The risks of radiation exposure and discomfort during the procedure should be considered in light of the benefits (Goldberg & Chavin, 1997). Research has shown that many patients have concerns related to risks from radiation and fear of pain during the procedure. Providing adequate teaching and support for these women as they participate in screening programs is essential to ensuring continued compliance with detection guidelines (Bakker, Lightfoot, Steggles, & Jackson, 1998).

Pharmacologic Prevention for Familial Breast Cancer

In 1998, the U.S. Food and Drug Administration approved the first drug ever indicated to reduce the incidence of cancer. The drug tamoxifen citrate, marketed by Zeneca Pharmaceuticals (Wilmington, DE) as Nolvadex®, has been shown in clinical trials to reduce breast cancer by 44% in women at high risk of developing the disease. Healthy women of all ages and at all levels of high risk of developing breast cancer have benefited from the therapy. In addition, women with atypical breast hyperplasia had an 88% reduction in incidence of invasive breast cancer. The drug is only indicated for prevention in women at high risk for developing the disease.

Healthcare providers can use the Gail Model Risk Assessment Tool to determine patients' appropriateness for tamoxifen citrate therapy. Healthcare professionals can obtain a Gail Model Risk Assessment Tool from Zeneca Pharmaceuticals by calling 800-34-Life4. Figure 2.4 lists the criteria for evaluating high-risk patients.

Prostate Cancer Screening

Screening practices for prostate cancer in asymptomatic men are controversial. Prostate cancer is the most prevalent malignancy among older men. More than 80% of patients diagnosed with prostate cancer are over 65 years old (O'Rourke & Germino, 1998). This disease actually has three forms: a latent form, which is not harmful; a progressive form, which can be fatal; and a rapidly progressive form, which is so malignant that the outcome is usually fatal despite early detection. Older men with the less-progressive form of prostate cancer may die of other causes before their cancer becomes evident. A diagnosis of prostate cancer in older men may lead to biopsy and aggressive treatment options that may not be necessary and may not prolong life. Treatment options supported by research include radical prostatectomy, radiation therapy, hormonal therapy, and "watchful waiting." Until national and international recommendations become uniform, providers should use a decision-making process that involves the older patient in making decisions regarding screening. Presence of other risk factors for prostate cancer beyond age should be weighed in the decision to pursue screening (Gerard & Frank-Stromborg, 1998). When considering screening practices, balancing treatment options with predictions of life expectancy may be complicated by lack of indicators of tumor aggressiveness as well as attitudes of providers toward aging that continue to influence cancer care (O'Rourke & Germino). General health-promotion recommendations advise men to use the following approach to prostate screening.

- Men under age 50 with no prostate symptoms should have an annual digital rectal exam (DRE).
- Men ages 50–75 should have the prostate-specific antigen (PSA) laboratory study in addition to the DRE.
- Men over age 75 may choose to omit the PSA screening.
- African Americans and those with family histories of prostate cancer may start PSA screening at younger ages.

Studies support a need for increased educational efforts related to detection practices among African American men, who have the highest incidence of and mortality rates for pros-

Figure 2.4. Criteria for Evaluating High Risk of Developing Breast Cancer

Age ≥ 35 years with history of lobular carcinoma in situ OR age ≥ 35 years with five-year predicted risk of breast cancer ≥ 1.67%, based on the following risk factors
- Number of first-degree relatives with breast cancer
- History and number of breast biopsies
- History of atypical hyperplasia
- Age at menarche
- Age at first live birth or nulliparity

Note. Based on information from Fisher et al., 1998.

tate cancer (Weinrich, Weinrich, Boyd, & Atkinson, 1998). A DRE should be performed by a healthcare provider who is skilled in recognizing subtle prostate abnormalities, including those of symmetry and consistency as well as marked induration or nodules. DRE is less effective in detecting prostate carcinoma than PSA (ACS, 1998).

Colorectal Cancer Screening

Screening practices for colorectal cancer have been criticized as being poorly supported by randomized studies. However, recent large studies on both sigmoidoscopy and fecal occult blood testing have shown a clear benefit to regular testing (Goldberg & Chavin, 1997). Individuals with a history of colorectal polyps, inflammatory bowel disease, Crohn's disease, or ulcerative colitis should consider increased frequency of screening and the addition of colonoscopy to detect lesions in the proximal bowel (Mahon, 1995). ACS has developed practitioner guidelines for the screening and surveillance necessary for early detection of colorectal polyps and cancer.

On the Horizon—Research on Screening

NCI is sponsoring a 10-year project called the Prostate, Lung, Colorectal, and Ovarian Screening Trial to determine the benefits and limitations of the screening tests used to detect these diseases. Volunteers will be randomized to an intervention or control group. The intervention group will receive chest x-rays and flexible sigmoidoscopy. Men will have a DRE and PSA screening. Women will have a pelvic exam, CA-125 testing, and transvaginal ultrasound. The control group will receive no special screening. All participants will be asked to complete a health questionnaire for up to 14 years. Information on this study, which began in 1998, can be found through NCI's Web site (http://dcp.nci.nih.gov/plco) or the NCI Cancer Information Service (800-4-CANCER). See Table 2.2 for ACS recommendations for the early detection of cancer in asymptomatic adults over 65 years of age.

Pharmaceuticals and Prevention

A clinical trial of the osteoporosis drug raloxifene (Evista®, Eli Lilly & Co., Indianapolis, IN) is showing promise as a preventative agent against breast cancer. Clinical trials of the drug show it is associated with a 55% reduction in the risk of breast cancer after three years of use. The clinical trials involved 10,575 women who have been followed for a median time of 40 months (Burton, 1998).

Molecular Genetic Technology

A relatively new and rapidly developing scientific body of knowledge that will become increasingly more important in cancer detection is molecular genetic technology. This testing involves analysis of human nucleic acids such as DNA and RNA, chromosomes, proteins, and metabolites that may determine cancer predisposition. Some older adults and, particularly, those with family histories of specific types of cancers may wish to seek genetic predisposition testing. Reliability of results, lack of quality-control procedures in laboratories, and varying costs are some of the problems surrounding this new technology. Oncology practitioners will need to become familiar with this technology and will need to be able to explain the results and implications to their clients. In most cases, a finding of predisposition should result in a heightened diligence in following the cancer screening protocols available to the individual (Loescher, 1998).

Table 2.2. American Cancer Society Recommendations for the Early Detection of Cancer in Asymptomatic Adults Over 65 Years of Age

Health Counseling and Cancer Check-Up	Population	Frequency
Breast self-examination	Women	Every month
Mammogram	Women	Every year
Clinical breast examination	Women	Every year
Endometrium	Women at high risk for endometrial cancer	Endometrial tissue sample at menopause
Pap test	Women	Every year; after three or more consecutive normal annual exams, may be less often at discretion of provider
Pelvic examination	Women	Every year
Fecal blood test	Men and women	Every year
Serum prostate-specific antigen and digital rectal examination (DRE)	Men	Every year (an abnormal test has been defined as a value above 4.0 mg/ml)
Flexible sigmoidoscopy and DRE*		Every five years
Colonoscopy and DRE*		Every 10 years
Double contrast barium enema and DRE*		Every 5–10 years

*The DRE should be performed at the same time as sigmoidoscopy, colonoscopy, or double-contrast barium enema.
Note. The colorectal screening should be performed more often if any of the following colorectal cancer risk factors exist.
- A personal history of colorectal cancer or adenomatous polyps
- A strong family history of colorectal cancer or polyps (cancer in a first-degree relative younger than 60 or in two first-degree relatives of any age
- A personal history of chronic inflammatory bowel disease
- Families with hereditary colorectal cancer syndromes (familial adenomatous polyposis and hereditary nonpolyposis colon cancer) (ACS, revised 7/1/98).

Nursing Implications to Improve Compliance With Screening Guidelines

A number of nursing implications must be incorporated into the care of the older adult population if screening practices are to be accepted and if patients are going to comply with the recommendations. A recent study demonstrated that many older adults are not certain about the major warning signs of cancer. More than half did not know the meaning of blood in a bowel movement or pain as a sign of possible cancer. The majority of individuals in the study did not know that increasing age was a major risk factor for cancer (Fitch et al., 1997).

Sensitive Physical Assessment

Physical assessment in older adults requires sensitivity and awareness of the common characteristics associated with aging. Assisting individuals in undressing may help them to relax and may reveal problems or pain caused by movement and specific positions. Symptoms that individuals may not recognize as important can be detected at this time. Examples may include skin lesions, pain, or discharge from the vagina or rectum. Older patients who are made to feel comfortable in the exam room may be more compliant with return visits. Examples include providing casual conversation in a caring manner, making sure that the room is warm (75°F), and providing a warm blanket. If older patients have to wait in the examination room for any length of time, inquire about their comfort. Many older individuals are uncomfortable lying flat on the examination table or in one position for any length of time. Changes related to osteoarthritis and osteoporosis are common. A pillow under the head and, perhaps, knees may be helpful. Another approach is to allow patients to sit upright until the examination actually begins. Always assist older patients when they change positions or move from the examining table. Postural hypotension and balance problems are common and may make falls a risk (Murray & Zentner, 1997). The practitioner's touch should convey concern and a caring attitude. Use the time spent assisting patients to undress and waiting for the examination to begin to educate them about practices that may decrease cancer risks as well as the guidelines for detection practices. Review the warning signs for cancer that should be reported to the healthcare practitioner.

Cultural Barriers to Screening

Assessing patients for any concerns, misconceptions, or fears related to detection practices is important so that these may be addressed and so that compliance can be increased. Research has shown that older patients may be less knowledgeable and less likely to participate in cancer screening. Specific groups of older adults, such as African Americans and immigrants, may face additional factors that lead to a decrease in participation in cancer screening. These factors may include poverty, lack of education, lack of cancer knowledge, and inaccessibility of healthcare delivery. Other common barriers to health screening, such as sensory impairment, language, and transportation issues, exist across all groups. Cultural values, beliefs, and attitudes may influence willingness to participate in cancer screening. Factors that may affect compliance with detection practices among older adults include race, religion, ethnic background, gender, socioeconomic status, and sexual orientation.

Variables that are specific to particular groups of older adults must be addressed by the practitioner who is encouraging compliance with screening guidelines. Screening programs will be more effective if they are developed by practitioners who hold fundamental respect and understanding for the validity of perspectives that differ from their own. The culturally sensitive and informed practitioner will be more likely to develop detection programs tailored to specific populations and groups (Kagawa-Singer, 1997).

Cancer Fatalism

Cancer fatalism, or the belief that death is inevitable when cancer is present, is another value that can impact negatively on willingness to follow cancer-detection guidelines (Powe, 1995). Cancer fatalism may be defined as fear, a feeling of predetermination, pessimism, and inevitability of death related to a cancer diagnosis. The need for practitioners to assess beliefs, perceptions, and attitudes of patients toward the cancer diagnosis is apparent if the concept of cancer fatalism is to be identified. This assessment is particularly critical when working with older patient populations, individuals from lower socioeconomic groups, and culturally diverse patient groups. Asking simple questions such as "What comes to mind when you hear the word *cancer*?" and "What does the diagnosis of cancer mean to you?" may help to identify feelings about cancer. The practitioner is then responsible for providing factual information in place of the misconceptions in a manner that individuals accept. A technique that may be helpful is the use of older people who are cancer survivors. These individuals can be recruited to distribute screening information and provide role models for other older people who have been assessed as having a fatalistic attitude about cancer (Phillips, 1995).

Conclusion

Detection Programs: Mechanisms to Promote Compliance and Utilization

Screening programs must provide testing that is safe, accepted, convenient, and economical. Techniques for disseminating information to older adults must be creative and extensive. The family must be included in educational programs directed toward detection practices as family members often assist with scheduling, transportation, and follow-up for the appropriate screening tests. Educational programs and screening in older adults may be better received if they are offered in proximity to the individuals' homes. Studies have shown that detection measures such as mammography are better accepted if conducted in comfortable, noninstitutional environments (Bakker et al., 1998). Options to remind participants about follow-up should be offered. A program that uses reminder phone calls will not work for individuals who do not have telephones. Older adults may prefer reminder postcards or personal visits from clinic employees or volunteers (Skinner et al., 1998).

Appropriate ways to reach older adults include educational programs and poster presentations in senior centers and residences, community television programs, and senior newspapers and newsletters discussing detection practices appropriate for older adults and listing warning signs of cancer. Personal follow-up and contact with healthcare workers can help to reinforce and clarify information that individuals need.

A simple and yet valuable mechanism to encourage compliance with prevention practices and screening guidelines is to communicate support for these practices in the older adult in an enthusiastic, committed manner (Fox, Roetzheim, & Kingston, 1997). Postscreening interviews should be conducted to answer questions and address concerns about the procedure and findings and to assess satisfaction with the screening program (Bakker et al., 1998). Healthcare workers must give clear information at this time regarding dates for return visits and future screening appointments.

Most significant is the need for older adults to understand that although their risk of cancer is high because of their advancing age, they can benefit through early-detection measures that can diagnose cancer when it is curable or more easily treated.

References

American Cancer Society. (1998). *Cancer facts and figures—1998*. Atlanta: Author.

American Cancer Society 1996 Advisory Committee on Diet, Nutrition, and Cancer Prevention. (1996). Guidelines on diet, nutrition, and cancer prevention: Reducing the risk of cancer with healthy food choices and physical activity. *CA: A Cancer Journal for Clinicians, 46*, 325–341.

Andresen, G.P. (1998). Assessing the older patient. *RN, 61*(3), 46–56.

Ashley, M.J., & Ferrence, R. (1994). Moderate drinking and health: The scientific evidence. *Contemporary Drug Problems, 21*, 1–204.

Bakker, D.A., Lightfoot, N.E., Steggles, S., & Jackson, C. (1998). The experience and satisfaction of women attending breast cancer screening. *Oncology Nursing Forum, 25*, 115–121.

Berendt, M.C. (1998). Alterations in nutrition. In J.K. Itano & K.N. Taoka (Eds.), *Core curriculum for oncology nursing* (3rd ed.) (pp. 223–257). Philadelphia: Saunders.

Blesch, K.S., & Prohaska, T.R. (1991). Cervical cancer screening in older women. *Cancer Nursing, 14*, 141–147.

Boyle, D.M. (1994). Realities to guide novel and necessary nursing care in geriatric oncology. *Cancer Nursing, 27*, 125–136.

Boyle, D.M. (1996). Cancer in the elderly: The forgotten minority. In C.M. Hogan (Ed.), *Issues in managing the oncology patient: A current reference and bibliography* (pp. 1–73). New York: Philips Healthcare Co.

Boyle, D.M., Engelking, C., Blesch, K.S., Dodge, J., Sana, L., & Weinrick, S. (1992). Oncology Nursing Society position paper on cancer and aging: The mandate for oncology nursing. *Oncology Nursing Forum, 19*, 913–933.

Burton, T.M. (1998, December 11). Lilly's Evista shows promise in cancer test. *The Wall Street Journal*, pp. A3–A6.

Chen, H.H., Tabar, L., Fagerberg, G., & Duffy, S.W. (1995). Effect of breast cancer screening after age 65. *Journal of Medical Screening, 2*(2), 118.

Cheng, K.K., & Day, N.E. (1996). Nutrition and esophageal cancer. *Cancer Causes and Control, 7*, 33–40.

Cohen, H.J. (1994). Biology of aging as related to cancer. *Cancer, 74*, 2092–2100.

Dausch, J.G., & Nixon, D.W. (1990). Garlic: A review of its relationship to malignant disease. *Preventive Medicine, 19*, 346–361.

Dickey, L.L. (1994). *Clinician's handbook of preventive services: Put prevention into practice.* Waldorf, MD: American Nurses Publishing.

Ebersole, P. (1998). Trends in care delivery models, *Geriatric Nursing, 19*, 6–7.

Fisher, B., Costantino, J.P., Wickerham, D.L., Redmond, C.H., Kavanah, M., Cronin, W.M., Vogel, V., Robidoux, A., Dimitrov, N., Atkins, J., Daly, M., Wieand, S., Tan-Chiu, E., Ford, L., & Wolmark, N. (1998). Tamoxifen for prevention of breast cancer: Report of the National Surgical Adjuvant Breast and Bowel Project P-1 study. *Journal of the National Cancer Institute, 90*, 1371–1388.

Fitch, M., Greenberg, M., Levstein, L., Muir, M., Plante, S., & King, E. (1997). Health promotion and early detection of cancer in older adults: Assessing knowledge about cancer. *Oncology Nursing Forum, 24*, 1743–1748.

Fox, S.A., Roetzheim, R.G., & Kingston, S. (1997). Barriers to cancer prevention in the older person. *Clinical Geriatric Medicine, 13*(1), 79–95.

Gerard, M.J., & Frank-Stromborg, M. (1998). Screening for prostate cancer in asymptomatic men: Clinical, legal, and ethical implications. *Oncology Nursing Forum, 25*, 1561–1569.

Goldberg, T.H., & Chavin, S.I. (1997). Preventive medicine and screening in older adults. *Journal of the American Geriatrics Society, 45*, 344–354.

Goodwin, J., Samet, J., Key, C., Humber, C., Kutvirt, D., & Hunt, C. (1986). Stage at diagnosis of cancer varies with the age of the patient. *Journal of the American Geriatrics Society, 34*, 20–26.

Harrison, R.A., Waterbor, J.W., Mulligan, S., Bernreuter, W.K., Han, S.Y., Stanley, R.J., & Rubins, E. (1997). Breast cancer detection rates by screening mammography in elderly women. *The Breast Journal, 3*, 331–336.

Hill, H.A., & Austin, H. (1996). Nutrition and endometrial cancer. *Cancer Causes and Control, 7*, 83–94.

Kagawa-Singer, M. (1997). Addressing issues for early detection and screening in ethnic populations. *Oncology Nursing Forum, 24*, 1705–1711.

List, N.D. (1992). Problems in cancer screening in the older patient. *Oncology, 6*(Suppl. 2), 25–30.

Loescher, L. (1998). DNA testing for cancer predisposition. *Oncology Nursing Forum, 25*, 1317–1327.

Mahon, S. (1995). Using brochures to educate the public about the early detection of prostate and colorectal cancer. *Oncology Nursing Forum, 22*, 1413–1415.

Mandelblatt, J.S., Wheat, M.E., Monane, M., Moshief, R.D., Hollenberg, J.P., & Tang, J. (1992). Breast cancer screening for elderly women with and without comorbid conditions. *Annals of Internal Medicine, 116*, 722–730.

Marshall, J.R., & Boyle, P. (1996). Nutrition and oral cancer. *Cancer Causes and Control, 7*, 101–112.

Messina, M., & Barnes, S. (1991). The roles of soy products in reducing risk of cancer. *Journal of the National Cancer Institute, 83*, 541–546.

Morrison, C.H., Olsen, S.J., & Ashley, B.W. (1998). Screening and early detection of cancer. In J.K. Itano & K.N. Taoka (Eds.), *Core curriculum for oncology nursing* (3rd ed.) (pp. 696–710). Philadelphia: Saunders.

Murray, R.B., & Zentner, J.P. (1997). *Health promotion strategies through the lifespan* (6th ed.). Stamford, CT: Appleton & Lange.

National Cancer Institute. (1997). *NCI/PDQ Physician statement: Screening of cancer* [Online]. Available: http://oncolink.upenn.edu/pdq [1998, October].

Oncology Nursing Society. (1998). Patients' bill of rights for quality cancer care. *Oncology Nursing Forum, 25,* 1301.

O'Rourke, M.E., & Germino, B.B. (1998). Prostate cancer treatment decisions: A focus group exploration. *Oncology Nursing Forum, 25,* 97–103.

Ouslander, J., & Beck, J. (1982). Defining the health problems of the elderly. *Annual Review of Public Health, 3,* 55–83.

Parker, S.L., Tong, T., Bolden, S., & Wingo, P.A. (1997). Cancer statistics, 1997. *CA: A Cancer Journal for Clinicians, 47,* 5–7.

Phillips, J.M. (1995). Commentary. *Oncology Nursing Forum, 22,* 1359.

Powe, B.D. (1995). Cancer fatalism among elderly Caucasians and African Americans. *Oncology Nursing Forum, 22,* 1355–1359.

Robinson, B., & Beghe, C. (1997). Cancer screening in the older patient. *Clinical Geriatric Medicine, 13,* 97–118.

Rubenstein, L.Z., & Nahas, R. (1998). Primary and secondary prevention strategies in the older adult. *Geriatric Nursing, 19*(1), 11–18.

Satariano, W.A., Belle, S.H., & Swanson, G.M. (1986). The severity of breast cancer at diagnosis: A comparison of age and extent of disease in black and white women. *American Journal of Public Health, 76,* 779–782.

Skinner, C.S., Sykes, R.K., Monsees, B.S., Andriole, B.S., Arfken, C.L., & Fischer, E.B. (1998). Learn, share, and live: Breast cancer education for older, urban, minority women. *Health Education Behaviors, 25*(1), 60–78.

Strohl, R.A. (1998). Nursing care of the client with cancer of the gastrointestinal tract. In J.K. Itano & K.N. Taoka (Eds.), *Core curriculum for oncology nursing* (3rd ed.) (pp. 460–480). Philadelphia: Saunders.

Teneriello, M.G., & Park, R.C. (1995). Early detection of ovarian cancer. *CA: A Cancer Journal for Clinicians, 45,* 71–87.

U.S. Department of Agriculture & U.S. Department of Health and Human Services. (1995). Nutrition and your health: Dietary guidelines for Americans (4th ed.). *Home and Garden Bulletin No. 232.* Washington, DC: U.S. Government Printing Office.

Weinrich, S.P., Weinrich, M.C., Boyd, M.D., & Atkinson, C. (1998). The impact of prostate cancer knowledge on cancer screening. *Oncology Nursing Forum, 25,* 527–534.

Zeigler, R.G., Mayne, S.T., & Swanson, C.A. (1996). Nutrition and lung cancer. *Cancer Causes and Control, 7,* 157–177.

Chapter Three

Interdisciplinary Management of the Older Adult With Cancer

Shirley S. Travis, PhD, RN, CS
Barbara Duer, BSN, RN

Introduction

Effectively managing the care of any patient involves interactions among formal providers (e.g., physicians, nurses, social workers, dietitians, therapists, chaplains), the patient, and the family. Historically, a noncollaborative approach was used in which the physician wrote the orders and others carried them out (Coyle, 1997). Although noncollaborative care may persist in some obscure healthcare situations, contemporary settings have either voluntarily adopted or been regulated to accept collaborative models as the better approach to patient care (Joint Commission on Accreditation of Healthcare Organizations, 1994). These models have been particularly well received in both oncology and gerontology practice settings where plans of care (1) tend to involve complex management regimens, (2) rely heavily on effective informal support systems, (3) span months or years, (4) cut across multiple levels, stages, or phases of care, (5) may not end in cure, (6) often include assistance at the end of life, and (7) are grossly ineffective without coordinated attention to the wholeness (mind, body, and spirit) of the person being treated.

The goal of this chapter is to integrate the art with the science of collaborative care for older adults with cancer. Our presentation of the science offers the reader a review of the structure and function of the two most commonly used collaborative models (interdisciplinary versus multidisciplinary) and some of the factors that have been associated with creating effective collaboration climates. In contrast, the art we seek to portray consists of the creative and imaginative ways practitioners must think about translating this information into meaningful and rewarding care in their organizations.

Multidisciplinary Versus Interdisciplinary Care

Whether the terms are teamwork, partnership, or collaboration, the intent in the new language of patient care is that successful patient outcomes require the vision and expert knowledge of many professionals working together with the patient and family to identify and achieve desired patient outcomes. In health care, providers tend to organize into one of two models of teaming: multidisciplinary or interdisciplinary. Although the terms are sometimes used interchangeably, these are two very different collaborative team models.

Multidisciplinary teams include members from several different disciplines who share common goals but work independently from one another to propose and implement patient interventions (Robertson, 1992; Tuchman, 1996). Multidisciplinary team members generally retain strong attachments to their discipline-specific knowledge and hold on to traditional roles and responsibilities. Regular communication among the members to achieve goals is not required, and team members operate with little or no integrated effort across disciplines (Tuchman). In contrast, interdisciplinary teams work together to identify and analyze problems, plan actions and interventions, and monitor results of the care plan. Team meetings are used to make or negotiate assignments, share information, and evaluate the team's effort toward achieving patient outcomes. Lines of communication among team members are highly visible, while disciplinary boundaries are purposely blurred (Robertson; Tuchman).

Because interdisciplinary teams seem to offer advantages over multidisciplinary teams for groups with complex problems, such as older adults with cancer, interdisciplinary teams are emphasized in this chapter (MacKinnon & Rae, 1996; Robertson, 1992). In many settings, however, multidisciplinary teams work extremely well as coordinating hubs for professionals of different disciplines. For example, programs with well-defined case management plans, groups developing acute-care critical pathways (often called multidisciplinary plans of care), care pathways, and certain discharge planning models are well suited to multidisciplinary approaches because the emphasis is on the individual competencies of the professional team members needed to achieve the desired patient outcomes in a timely fashion (Closs, Ferguson, & Thompson, 1996; Holt, 1997; Lynn-McHale, Fitzpatrick, & Shaffer, 1993; Nugent, 1992)

Unfortunately, simply bringing representatives from many disciplines together does not ensure that they will function effectively (Robertson, 1992). In fact, several factors are known to work against collaborative models, in general, and interdisciplinary teams, in particular. These factors include outdated hierarchical structures among healthcare providers, "turf" issues, discipline allegiances to the exclusion of collaborative efforts, and role conflicts (Castledine, 1996; Perkins & Tryssenaar, 1994). We will return to these barriers throughout the chapter.

Creating Effective Interdisciplinary Teams

The ways in which healthcare professionals are educated in the United States and elsewhere generally are not conducive to an interdisciplinary spirit or philosophy of shared patient care. Although interdisciplinary collaborative practice opportunities are receiving increasing support while students are in school, the truly revolutionary changes in traditional teaching methods that will be needed to affect collaborative behavior over the long term have been slow to develop (Clark, 1997; Cunningham, 1997; Larson, 1995). Consequently, the educational systems that should socialize new health professionals into their roles persist in preparing professionals who do not know what is needed to create effective interdisciplinary teams and have not had the opportunity to develop skill in collaborative critical thinking. As a result, when professionals find themselves in collaborative-practice environments, they must be given time to make the conceptual shift from being providers in traditional hierarchical relationships to becoming caregiving partners on empowering teams (Clark; Felten, Cady, Metzler, & Burton, 1997; Larson; Wesorick, 1997).

Organizations that have developed effective collaborative models for interdisciplinary practice report very similar sets of factors necessary to ensure success. Perhaps above all else, a collaborative mindset must prevail that views collaboration as an opportunity and that gives players "permission" to cross traditional boundaries (Liedtka & Whitten, 1997). As Wesorick (1997) discussed, the development of care partners also must be accompanied by personal choice to enter into the collaborative arrangement; organization clarity and support for the work of the partners; equal accountability among the partners for the team's success; the potential for all team members to learn, grow, and create harmonious relationships on the team; and personal trust among the partners that creates a "flow of energy between all the principles" (p. 7).

Clearly, requirements for effective teaming cannot be mandated by organizational policy or procedure, nor can one player force others to embrace interdisciplinary ideals. Team members often need to work on clarifying their goals for interdisciplinary teaming, learn to be open and effective communicators, and appreciate the contributions of each member in achieving patient outcomes (Antai-Otong, 1997; Miaskowski, Jacox, Hester, & Ferrell, 1992). In the absence of any prior knowledge or skill in effective interdisciplinary teaming, the team will likely go through several developmental stages before it performs at its maximal level of efficiency and effectiveness (Antai-Otong). Something as simple as finding a mutually convenient time and location to meet for regular team meetings can be stressful to fledgling interdisciplinary teams.

The Membership of Interdisciplinary Teams

The choice of which disciplines to include on the interdisciplinary team should take into consideration the unique characteristics of the patients and families being served, such as social, economic, or cultural variation, as well as the core of common problems and needs that the team must address. Typically, a core team in health care consists of one representative from medicine, one from nursing, and one from social work. Then, as the needs of individual patients dictate the need for additional members, representatives from other disciplines are invited to team meetings. As outlined by Robertson (1992), the advantages of a small team are that the members have fewer interpersonal issues to address to become a working team, can more easily focus on the issues, and have fewer logistical problems with meeting dates and times. Also, when teams are small, the organization spends fewer personnel dollars on time spent in meetings. The most obvious disadvantage in selecting a small core team is that the plan of care is drastically limited to the skill and expertise of the core disciplines. Professionals who should be involved in all aspects of the patient's plan of care have fewer opportunities to participate in developing and implementing an integrated plan.

For a variety of reasons, the leaders of interdisciplinary teams are either physicians, nurses (often advanced practice nurses involved in patient care), or social workers. No empirical evidence suggests that these professionals make the best team leaders. Rather, the choice of who will keep the work of the team on track should be made based on who is in the best coordinating position within the organization and who is the most effective group leader. Discipline membership is a weak selection criterion for a group leader.

Oncology care now occurs in inpatient, ambulatory care, and home- and community-based care settings and includes the multitude of services often referred to as supportive care services (Cornelius, 1997). Consequently, the composition of interdisciplinary team membership can and should vary. As shown in Figure 3.1, if desired outcomes vary across settings and service types and certain mixes of professionals are better at achieving the desired outcomes than other mixes, then achieving the diverse outcomes of oncology care requires some variation of interdisciplinary team membership. Moreover, if the desired outcome requires highly specialized knowledge, such as pain management or other complex symptom management (see Chapters 9 and 10), more than one team may be needed in a setting. Decisions about when to integrate and when to segregate interdisciplinary teams should be made on the basis of outcomes. Desired and achievable patient outcomes should drive the choices about who to include on the interdisciplinary teams and how many different teams an organization needs, rather than having a predefined pattern of interdisciplinary work limit the outcomes of care.

Interdisciplinary Team Membership Across Supportive Care Services

Supportive care services are those medical and psychosocial services that promote and enhance quality of life by focusing on the whole person within his or her family system (Coluzzi & Rhiner, 1996). Despite efforts by the National Cancer Institute (NCI) to standardize the array of supportive services available to patients with cancer, no single taxonomy of services has been established. As conceptualizations of these services continue to be developed, refined, and interpreted into an accepted standard of care, many leading authorities on the topic have settled on the inclusion of both curative and noncurative care (active palliation and palliative care) in the general oncologic model of care (Coluzzi et al., 1995).

The primary goals of those teams with responsibility for curative therapy are plans for the reversal of the disease process and prolongation of life with secondary goals of symptom control (Coluzzi & Rhiner, 1996). In contrast, active palliation and hospice teams focus on the control of symptoms and support the patient and family to achieve their goals. Consistent with the noncurative foci, these latter teams also work to promote and enhance the quality of life of patients living with cancer (Leland & Schonwetter, 1997).

The most frequently offered personal support services at NCI-designated cancer centers, in descending order, are dietary support, ostomy care, rehabilitation services, sexual counseling, and specialized pain management (Coluzzi et al., 1995). Given the earlier discussion of core team membership on interdisciplinary management teams, these model cancer centers obviously cannot operate effectively with limited core team memberships. In fact, in one clinical model for hospice care of a patient who was terminally ill, Coluzzi and Rhiner (1996) identified 10 key members of the team: the patient, friends, family members, volunteers, chaplain, social worker, nurse, medical director, attending physician, and home health aides. This team configuration is contrasted with their clinical model for pain management, which includes the

Figure 3.1. The Reasoning Behind Variable Interdisciplinary Teams

- If desired outcomes vary across setting and service types, and certain mixes of professionals are better at achieving certain outcomes than other mixes, then the membership of interdisciplinary teams must vary.

patient, family members, friends, psychologist, rehabilitation specialist, social worker, clinical nurse specialist, physician pain specialist, medical oncologist, chaplain, and pharmacist. Although the essential elements of supportive care services are not yet identified, the tripartite core of supportive care—patient choice, collaboration, and interdisciplinary models—appears to be firmly established and widely accepted in cancer care. Thus, discussions of interdisciplinary teams for aging patients with cancer must be broad and include an array of teams with goals ranging from anticancer treatments/curative therapy to active palliation and palliative/hospice care; all of which require an adequate mix of team members to achieve the care goals.

Interdisciplinary Knowledge Is "New" Knowledge

One of the serendipitous, or unexpected, results of interdisciplinary teaming can be the opportunity for team members to create "new" knowledge at the points where existing knowledge from their individual disciplinary perspectives converge on patient problems and needs. Beyond simply sharing information or influencing another team member's point of view, interdisciplinary collaboration creates interdisciplinary knowledge (McHugh et al., 1996). For example, the concept of functionality (the ability to care for oneself and to get around in daily living) in the gerontology literature means different things to the separate disciplines of nursing, rehabilitation therapy, medicine, social work, and clinical psychology, to name a few. But, when an interdisciplinary plan is applied to the problems and needs of clients with functional decline, team actions include richer, more finely focused, better coordinated, and more comprehensive qualities than actions that are segregated by disciplinary boundaries. The team addresses the whole person in decline rather than separating the person into disciplinary compartments.

In the next sections, some of the issues that interdisciplinary team members must consider in providing developmentally appropriate cancer care to older adults will be described. Because other chapters address specific care issues, this chapter focuses on the more general knowledge of adult development and aging that all team members should understand.

Providing Developmentally Appropriate Care to Older Adults

Cancer, when first diagnosed and confirmed, forces the patient and family to make a multitude of difficult decisions, including treatment choice, the preferred locations of treatment and care, and methods of symptom management (Lewis, Pearson, Corcoran-Perry, & Narayan, 1997). The interdisciplinary team stands ready to provide the education and information needed and to enact the selected plan of care. In the broadest sense, this cancer-care scenario is no different for patients of any age. The critical difference is in the ability of the organization to provide appropriate care that considers all aspects of human development (biological, psychosocial, spiritual) and the characteristics of the patient's available social support network (Boyle et al., 1992).

With developmentally appropriate care in mind, we also understand that the older adult with cancer comes to the interdisciplinary team with a variety of life experiences that very likely include prior exposure to acute and chronic illness. This is not to say that all older people have disabling chronic illness or that disease is a normal part of aging. In fact, for the vast majority (60%) of older adults who report any chronic illness, the conditions do not significantly limit their daily activities (Freudenheim, 1996). The point is that older adults, unlike many of their younger patient counterparts, often have given some thought to the actual or potential impact of disease on their lives, quality-of-life issues, and end-of-life preferences prior to the time when the cancer diagnosis is made.

Biological Issues

Human beings are continuously changing, adapting, and responding to the maturing bodies in which they live. From a biological perspective, both normal physiologic aging changes and changes confounded by the pathophysiology of disease affect the physical condition of older people. Aggressive cancer treatment may not be a good choice for older patients with significant comorbidity and functional decline because they may not survive the toxic effects of chemotherapy or radiation (Boyle, 1994). Therefore, the interdisciplinary team will need to consider the effects of normal and pathologic processes of aging and base treatment options on physiologic data regarding the body's ability to respond to treatment. Decisions are not based solely on the individual's age.

Virtually every system in the body undergoes normal age-related changes. Many of these changes have a considerable effect on the absorption, distribution, metabolism, and excretion of antineoplastic agents (Boyle, 1994). In addition, chemotherapy may stress or damage aged body systems that are functioning effectively but that have reduced buffer zones between compensated and uncompensated conditions. Unfortunately, unlike pediatric oncology, few guidelines for geriatric dose titration of antineoplastic agents are available (Boyle). Thus, the interdisciplinary team must closely monitor the patient for adverse responses to the chemotherapy.

A confounding factor in the treatment of older adults is a history of medication use. Pre-existing self-medication practices with over-the-counter medications and prescribed medications for chronic conditions can complicate the plan of care. Because the treatment of other conditions will not and should not cease during the cancer treatment, a consulting geriatrician or clinical pharmacist may be a vital part of a team that is managing complicated medication regimens. Teasing apart the causes of adverse drug reactions such as confusion, dizziness, nausea, and vomiting becomes extraordinarily complex when dealing with older adults whose physiological responses and drug interaction pictures can be anything but "textbook." Finally, because older adults are vulnerable to undertreatment of or failure to treat coexisting conditions when a chronic illness is being treated, the interdisciplinary team should remain vigilant for seemingly unrelated problems that can affect a patient's well being and quality of life, including arthritis pain or the need for hormone replacement therapy (Redelmeier, Tan, & Booth, 1998).

Psychosocial Issues

Investigations of the psychology and sociology of adult development and aging attempt to explain how individual behavior and the lives of individuals become organized (or disorganized) as they age (Ferraro, 1990). Studying psychosocial development includes such constructs and concepts as life events, cohort membership, role enactment, self-concept, intelligence, and personality.

Understanding the complex life histories and multitude of choices that people make as they age is beyond the scope of most healthcare interactions. As a result, healthcare providers have come to use the construct of subjective well-being as a proxy for an individual's intellectual and emotional assessment of life as a whole. This global measure is believed to represent at least four different aspects of well-being: (1) the degree to which a person has attained desired goals, (2) long-term happiness with life, (3) transient feelings of pleasure, and (4) transient feelings of distress, such as anxiety, depression, and worry (Liang & Whitelaw, 1990). Measuring a patient's subjective well-being is important because it can be a powerful predictor of the success of an intervention program, an important marker of patient improvement or decline during the course of treatment, and a useful outcome measure in combination with traditional survival and biomedical parameters (Liang & Whitelaw).

Interdisciplinary teams that work with older adults can and should seek convenient, quantifiable measures of subjective well-being. But developing an effective plan of care is virtually impossible without some understanding of the complex psychosocial life histories that older adults and their significant others bring to cancer treatment programs. Teams often collect this information in bits and pieces over time. More developmentally adept teams will have a significant amount of this information at the onset of the care planning process. Important information can be efficiently obtained without spending hours collecting a life history. A series of short open-ended questions might include the following. "What were the four or five most important or meaningful decisions you have made in your life?" "Overall, how do you feel about the decisions and choices you have made?" "Describe a stressful time in your life, and tell me how you and your family handled the situation."

Spiritual Issues

Spirituality is the term generally applied to a person's connectedness with life, living, and the environment beyond oneself. A person's meaning and purpose in life is derived from spirituality. It also empowers individuals to be integrated wholes and to experience life fully (Fehring, Miller, & Shaw, 1997). Religiosity, in contrast, describes the ways in which people express their religious beliefs and practices. Religiosity and spirituality are related to three other important constructs in cancer care: hope, effective coping, and quality of life (Fehring et al.). See Chapter 12 for an in-depth discussion of spiritual care of the older adult with cancer.

One common misconception about aging is that as people age, their religion becomes an increasingly significant part of the adult development and aging experience. For many older people, religion is an important way of expressing spirituality and keeping them connected to a social community. However, religion is not required for personal spirituality. This is an important distinction to make because, although the interdisciplinary team may not feel competent to address religiosity, the team must be concerned with the patient's spirituality and connections to hope, coping, quality of life, and the desired end-of-life experience (Herth, 1989).

For example, hopeless or depressed people are not only difficult to work with, but they also can instill hopelessness in those around them, including their formal and informal caregivers. A vicious cycle can begin in which caregivers withdraw from the discomforting relationship and subsequently withhold needed support services, exacerbating the care recipient's hopelessness (Barnard, 1995; Miller & Oertel, 1992). One effective intervention for hopelessness is the application of early and continuous support resources for the individual's spiritual well-being. Thus, the intervention bolsters the patient's intrinsic abilities to cope with the cancer experience (Fehring et al., 1997). Although a chaplain or other spiritual advisor is often part of or available to interdisciplinary teams working with older patients with cancer, religion and spirituality are not synonymous. Effective interventions for spiritual well-being must be interdisciplinary and not just something the chaplain deals with.

Families and Other Informal Support Issues

Regardless of the patient's age, several types of family-focused support often are needed: informational, anticipatory guidance, interpretive guidance, skill-based information, problem-focused services, and physical services (Lewis, 1990). Part of every interdisciplinary team assessment process should be a family assessment of the problems and needs of the family unit as it enters cancer care.

A common misconception is that older people do not have adequate family or social support networks to support their caregiving needs. In reality, the personal networks of older adults include a significant proportion of both family and friends (Antonucci & Akiyama, 1995), many of whom could be called upon to support cancer care. One obvious difference between the families and social supports of older adult patients and those of their younger counterparts lies in the structure and function of significant supporting relationships. Perhaps the most widely used and highly regarded conceptual model for studying social relations in old age is the convoys model of social support. According to the model, people form social relationships and move through their lifetimes surrounded by individuals who are close and important to them and who have a critical influence on their lives and well-being (Antonucci & Akiyama). A special feature of these older adult relationships is the accumulation of feelings and emotions (positive and negative) that accompany long-term associations and constantly changing relationships.

When interdisciplinary teams work with family members and significant others of older patients, they should be prepared for the complex relational histories they will discover during these encounters. For example, spouses who have been married 50 or more years have relationships that are built on a long history of shared interests, values, and affection. An understanding of the unaffected spouse's feelings, fears, and uncertainty about the future is not possible without some appreciation of the couple's relational history. Similarly, siblings of advanced age, especially those who have maintained close geographic proximity and life circumstances, typically express strong feelings of solidarity when faced with a family or personal crisis, such as a sibling with cancer (Circirelli, 1989). Team members must understand that in the absence of or in addition to a spouse or adult children, siblings often are powerful support people for older adult patients.

In general, interactions with friends are thought to be used for pleasure, whereas family interactions are suitable for daily needs, including caregiving tasks. These relationship functions can change when older adults need assistance with chronic or long-term care (Travis, 1995). Less understood is whether a similar reliance on friends occurs with cancer care. Widowhood, geographic distance of adult children and other relatives, and changes in family size, configuration, and the availability of family caregivers may create greater reliance on friends in the future. This is an area of oncology/gerontology care that requires additional research.

Goal-Directed Interdisciplinary Care for Older Adults With Cancer

Through most of this chapter, the authors have suggested that the primary purpose of interdisciplinary oncology teams is to address an array of patient and family problems and needs that require interdisciplinary action to achieve desired outcomes. This message actually is not consistent with the newer approaches to gerontology/geriatrics care planning that are being used in some healthcare settings. More recent approaches to care are based on goal-directed rather than problem-oriented plans of care and include the patient and family as the primary decision makers in deciding which problems or needs will be addressed in goal-directed care (Mold, 1995). Among those oncology teams that provide noncurative care to older adults with cancer, many aged patients come to these teams with problems and needs (some long-standing and some chronic) that they neither expect nor want the team to address during their extended care.

The newer emphasis on goal-directed care is consistent with several points that have been made in this chapter. First, with goal-directed care, the composition of the interdisciplinary team must be flexible enough to accommodate the array of goals that patients and their families may select. Traditional approaches to care planning do not work when patients are empowered to decide on the relative importance of a set of problems and needs and to decide which concerns they want to resolve. Second, although some patient goals may be short term and relatively simple to achieve with discipline-specific interventions, most goals for older patients with cancer will be complex and require more long-term interventions that are best served by interdisciplinary action plans. Finally, a focus on goal-directed care shifts the focus from trying to minimize problems or deficits to maximizing the patient's strengths and potential; this is a paradigm shift that requires collaborative teamwork (Mold, 1995).

Conclusion

Collaborative practice is not unique to oncology or gerontology/geriatrics. However, this chapter addresses why interdisciplinary teaming, in particular, is well suited to the care of older adults with cancer. As life expectancies increase and more adults enter the last stage of life healthy and fit, cancer care for older adults will continue to evolve. Interdisciplinary care will change and mature as the depth, breadth, art, and science of that care is clarified and articulated. To this end, a great deal of additional work is needed to refine collaborative practice models, delineate the essential elements of developmentally appropriate care for older adults, challenge prevailing myths of aging that may be affecting cancer care for older adults, and create "new" knowledge for interdisciplinary practice.

References

Antai-Otong, D. (1997). Team building in a health care setting. *American Journal of Nursing, 97*(7), 48–51.

Antonucci, T.C., & Akiyama, H. (1995). Convoys of social relations: Family and friendships within a life span context. In R. Blieszner & V. Bedford (Eds.), *Handbook of aging and the family* (pp. 355–371). Westport, CT: Greenwood Press.

Barnard, D. (1995). Chronic illness and the dynamics of hoping. In S.K. Toombs, D. Barnard, & R.A. Carson (Eds.), *Chronic illness* (pp. 39–57). Bloomington, IN: Indiana University Press.

Boyle, D.M. (1994). Realities to guide novel and necessary nursing care in geriatric oncology. *Cancer Nursing, 17,* 125–136.

Boyle, D.M., Engelking, C., Blesch, K.S., Dodge, J., Sarna, L., & Weinrich, S. (1992). Oncology Nursing Society position paper on cancer and aging: The mandate for oncology nursing. *Oncology Nursing Forum, 19,* 913–933

Castledine, G. (1996). Encouraging team collaboration in healthcare. *British Journal of Nursing, 5,* 1402.

Circirelli, V.G. (1989). Feelings of attachment to siblings and well-being in later life. *Psychology and Aging, 4,* 211–216.

Clark, P.G. (1997). Values in health care professional socialization: Implications for geriatric education in interdisciplinary teamwork. *The Gerontologist, 37,* 441–451.

Closs, S.J., Ferguson, A., & Thompson, D. (1996). Collaborating on the integration of cancer nursing services. *Nursing Standard, 10*(50), 37–40.

Coluzzi, P., Grant, M., Doroshow, J., Rhiner, M., Ferrell, B., & Rivera, L. (1995). Survey of the provision of supportive care services at National Cancer Institute-designated cancer centers. *Journal of Clinical Oncology, 13,* 756–764.

Coluzzi, P.H., & Rhiner, M. (1996). Supportive care services. In R. McCorkle, M. Grant, M. Frank-Stromborg, & S.B. Baird (Eds.), *Cancer nursing: A comprehensive textbook* (2nd ed.) (pp. 1322–1332). Philadelphia: Saunders.

Cornelius, F. (1997). Homecare, alternative care settings, and cancer resources. In S. Otto (Ed.), *Oncology nursing* (pp. 679–711). St. Louis: Mosby.

Coyle, N. (1997). Interdisciplinary collaboration in hospital palliative care: Chimera or goal? *Palliative Medicine, 11,* 265–266.

Cunningham, W.F. (1997). Post graduate education for general practitioners: Interdisciplinary education would help improve teamwork. *British Medical Journal, 315,* 1543.

Fehring, R.J., Miller, J.F., & Shaw, C. (1997). Spiritual well-being, religiosity, hope, depression, and other mood states in elderly people coping with cancer. *Oncology Nursing Forum, 24,* 663–671.

Felten, S., Cady, N., Metzler, M.H., & Burton, S. (1997). Implementation of collaborative practice through interdisciplinary rounds on a general surgery service. *Nursing Case Management, 2,* 122–126.

Ferraro, K.F. (1990). Sociology of aging: The micro-macro link. In K.F. Ferraro (Ed.), *Gerontology: Perspectives and issues* (pp. 110–128). New York: Springer.

Freudenheim, E. (1996). *Chronic care in America: A 21ˢᵗ century challenge.* Princeton, NJ: Robert Wood Johnson Foundation.

Herth, D.A. (1989). The relationship between level of hope and level of coping response and other variables in patients with cancer. *Oncology Nursing Forum, 16,* 67–72.

Holt, F.M. (1997). Do we need a report card for interdisciplinary collaboration? *Clinical Nurse Specialist, 11,* 133.

Joint Commission on Accreditation of Healthcare Organizations. (1994). *Accreditation manual for hospitals.* Chicago: Author.

Larson, E.L. (1995). New rules for the game: Interdisciplinary education for health professionals. *Nursing Outlook, 43,* 180–185.

Leland, J.Y., & Schonwetter, R.S. (1997). Advances in hospice care. *Clinics in Geriatric Medicine, 13,* 381–399.

Lewis, F.M. (1990). Strengthening family supports. *Cancer, 65,* 752–759.

Lewis, M., Pearson, V., Corcoran-Perry, S., & Narayan, S. (1997). Decision making by elderly patients with cancer and their caregivers. *Cancer Nursing, 20,* 389–397.

Liang, J., & Whitelaw, N.A. (1990). Assessing the physical and mental health of the elderly. In S.M. Stahl (Ed.), *The legacy of longevity* (pp. 35–54). Thousand Oaks, CA: Sage.

Liedtka, J., & Whitten, E. (1997). Building better patient care services: A collaborative approach. *Health Care Management Review, 22,* 16–24.

Lynn-McHale, D.J., Fitzpatrick, E.R., & Shaffer, R.B. (1993). Case management: Development of a model. *Clinical Nurse Specialist, 7,* 299–307.

MacKinnon, J.L., & Rae, N.M. (1996). Fostering geriatric interdisciplinary collaboration through academic education. *Physical and Occupational Therapy in Geriatrics, 14,* 41–49.

McHugh, M., West, P., Assatly, C., Duprat, L., Howard, L., Niloff, J., Waldo, K., Wandel, J., & Clifford, J. (1996). Establishing an interdisciplinary patient care team: Collaboration at the bedside and beyond. *Journal of Nursing Administration, 26*(4), 21–27.

Miaskowski, C., Jacox, A., Hester, N.O., & Ferrell, B. (1992). Interdisciplinary guidelines for the management of acute pain: Implications for quality improvement. *Journal of Nursing Quality Care, 7*(1), 1–6.

Miller, J.F., & Oertel, C.B. (1992). Powerlessness in the elderly: Preventing hopelessness. In J.F. Miller (Ed.), *Coping with chronic illness: Overcoming powerlessness* (pp. 135–160). Philadelphia: F.A. Davis.

Mold, J.W. (1995). An alternative conceptualization of health and health care: Its implications for geriatrics and gerontology. *Educational Gerontology, 21,* 85–101.

Nugent, K.E. (1992). The clinical nurse specialist as case manager in a collaborative practice model: Bridging the gap between quality and cost of care. *Clinical Nurse Specialist, 6,* 106–111.

Perkins, J., & Tryssenaar, J. (1994). Making interdisciplinary education effective for rehabilitation students. *Journal of Allied Health, 23,* 133–141.

Redelmeier, D.A., Tan, S.H., & Booth, G.L. (1998). The treatment of unrelated disorders in patients with chronic medical diseases. *New England Journal of Medicine, 338,* 1516–1520.

Robertson, D. (1992). The roles of health care teams in care of the elderly. *Family Medicine, 24,* 136–141.

Travis, S.S. (1995). Families and formal networks. In R. Blieszner & V. Bedford (Eds.), *Handbook of aging and the family* (pp. 459–473). Westport, CT: Greenwood Press.

Tuchman, L.I. (1996). The team and models of teaming. In P. Rosin, A. Whitehead, L.I. Tuchman, G.S. Jesien, A.L. Begun, & L. Irwin (Eds.), *Partnerships in family-centered care* (pp. 119–143). Baltimore: Paul Brookes Publishing.

Wesorick, B. (1997). Partnering: The invisible field of hope, potential and discovery for the work setting. *Creative Nursing, 3*(1), 1, 4–8.

Chapter Four

Home Management of the Older Adult With Cancer

Sue E. Meiner, EdD, RN, CS, GNP

Introduction

Cancer as a chronic disease is a relatively new concept in health care. As advances in technology and the treatment of cancers have continued over the past several decades, many forms of cancer now lead to drastically increased survival times. Current estimates suggest that a family member in three out of every four families will experience cancer during his or her lifetime. The increase in survival times and course of illness expand the number of months to years in which people are living at home with cancer diagnoses.

Otto (1995) noted that many elderly patients with cancer want to be at home with family and in familiar surroundings for as long as possible, with most wanting to die at home. She found that most family members feel inadequate about providing proper care to the patient with cancer. In addition, family caregivers may experience difficulty in meeting the continuing needs of other family members during intense times of caregiving.

Family-centered nursing has been a long-established practice focus. Considering the family as a unit further supports the homecare management of patients with cancer. When one member of a family is diagnosed with cancer, the entire family is affected. Corbin and Strauss (1988) noted that each family member makes adaptations to the one member's chronic illness that directly affect the day-to-day management of the chronic condition.

Influence of Gender and Marital Status on Cancer in the Elderly

Landis, Murray, Bolden, and Wingo's (1998) report on the National Cancer Institute's Surveillance, Epidemiology, and End Results Program of 1997, which provided statistics on gender and the probability of people developing invasive cancers between the ages of 60 and 79, found that men were at higher risk for all major categories of cancers except breast cancer. The lung cancer ratio was 1 in 15 for men and 1 in 26 for women. Colon and rectal cancer developed in approximately 1 in 24 men and 1 in 31 women. When all sites of cancer occurrence were statistically reviewed, older men were found to have invasive cancer at a ratio of one in two, while the ratio for older women was one in three.

These statistics partly explain the increased percentage of older women in the American population. Widowhood is an overwhelming reality for women over age 75. Elderly men tend to be married (American Association of Retired Persons, 1998). This feminization of the older population often means that women are without social or personal support in the home if a cancer diagnosis is made. As a result, when men are diagnosed with cancer, home care is possible in most cases with regular nursing monitoring, intermittent assistance with nursing care tasks, and a program of basic nursing care instruction to the caregiver in the household. However, widows living alone cannot take advantage of home care unless self-care is possible. When assisted living is required, these women need to find someone to help or relocate to a place where care can be provided.

Caregivers

Depending on patients' health status, financial conditions, and availability of significant others for support prior to the cancer diagnosis, elderly patients with cancer must decide on short-term and continuing living and care arrangements. Maintaining life at home should be the goal for the family and supported by healthcare providers. Nurses play a major role in providing the means and knowledge to help elderly patients stay at home as long as possible, even until death.

According to Hileman, Lackey, and Hassanein (1992), the number of family caregivers is rising annually because of cancer's changing prognoses. Technological improvements have made many forms of cancer chronic conditions. With lengths of illness changing and more cancer care being provided at home, identification of home caregiver needs is a priority for nursing interventions.

When family members are available to provide home-based care for loved ones with cancer, the family dynamics undergo considerable change. Decisions must be made regarding the primary caregiver. The family must decide who will be responsible for associated healthcare needs, such as transportation to the primary-care provider's office or clinic and obtaining necessary healthcare supplies and medications.

Caring for a terminally ill older adult often does not fit within a working family's life pattern. In other situations, no family members live nearby or can care for the elderly patient. When circumstances cannot support home care of elderly patients with cancer, institutional care must be found.

Psychosocial Impact on the Patient

Lueckenotte (1996) stated, "Because of its catastrophic nature, the diagnosis of cancer is a disease that almost universally generates feelings of stress in the individual on confirmation of the diagnosis" (p. 360). A sense of being isolated from family, friends, and activities often accompanies a cancer diagnosis in older people. These feelings may not be self-induced but result from the negativity of significant others who fear the disease.

Casual relationships frequently are broken off following disclosure of a cancer diagnosis. This avoidance behavior is thought to be associated with unresolved or personal feelings about death and dying and often suggests a fear of experiencing a profound loss.

Family Response to Terminal Illness

Patients and family members often experience shock following disclosure of a cancer diagnosis. After initial feelings of disbelief, family members frequently hold discussions about the future away from the patient. When uncomfortable feelings surround a diagnosis, the patient often is left out of discussions. Frequently, family members experience anticipatory grief. In an effort to cope with a problem-focused style, some family members may begin discussing options for living arrangements and care before understanding the prognosis and available treatment options (Chapman & Pepler, 1998). Nurses can provide meaningful assistance to these families by helping them to understand the meaning of the diagnosis to each member and the patient in an attempt to come to terms with a future that is unclear at best. The desires of the patient are paramount to any arrangements that family members might make collectively or individually.

Faced with everyday stresses, some families can become dysfunctional if adequate support is not present (Jassak, 1992). Even when families respond with resilience to the stresses of caring for the patient with cancer at home, diminished emotional and physical energy may result. Nurses can promote effective coping by helping family members gather strength from each other toward decision making. The goals of nursing in home care include providing psychological support aimed at achieving a successful pattern of adaptation by members of the family.

The Rally-Around Family Response

In some family groups, adversity and tragedy bring everyone together for strength and consolation. Decisions are made in an orderly manner and with agreement toward duties and responsibilities for current and future family needs. The patient is an integral part of the planning. In other family groups, the oldest adult child is expected to assume the caregiver role when the parents enter old age or if catastrophic illness occurs. Other family members wait for instructions for specific participation in the caregiving scenario.

When patients with cancer survive beyond what is expected, families may lose their focus on caregiving responsibilities. This uncertainty produces additional stress on both families and caregivers. Nurses must provide additional support during these times. One supportive technique has been to encourage family members to continue with their schedules of assistance while taking each day at a time. This can help the family to concentrate on the present pattern of caregiving instead of expending energy on worry about days or weeks in the future.

Failing Family Response

Other families do not respond with organization and distribution of responsibilities. Family members' chaotic expression of passing on duties and responsibilities to someone else is an overriding theme of every discussion, if they communicate at all. Adversity makes a weak relationship weaker. In this case, the nurse's role is to help the patient with securing services that will replace the loss of family relationships. Although replacing relationships is rarely fulfilling, the reassurance of someone being available when needed can reduce the anxiety of isolation.

Financial Strain

Older patients often discuss financial burdens and the ongoing drain on resources. This concern is frequently the basis for their treatment decisions. Elderly patients frequently express comments that their lives will soon be over and they should save for the younger family members rather than waste money that had been saved during earlier, productive years.

Family members view the burden of healthcare costs as differently as the reaction to the diagnosis. Some families pull together and pool resources for treatment options. Some will postpone vacations, home improvements, or leisure purchases to maintain emergency funds for care. Some apply for financial help from welfare agencies in lieu of using personal funds when treatment options exceed elderly patients' insurance benefits. Family dynamics can cause a delay or cancellation of treatment options if information is not readily available. Nurses should begin proactive interventions when the medical team prescribes a treatment plan. Close communication with the physician will be necessary to initiate interventions quickly.

The Impact of Physical Functioning on the Patient and Family

Self-care should be encouraged for as long as the patient's health status remains stable. Nurses can provide physical care in the home setting at intervals that allow the patient to perform as much self-care as possible. When self-care is being accomplished, nurses should help the patients to set goals that will permit adjustments as health needs change.

When self-care begins to become difficult and several activities of daily living (e.g., bathing, eating, toileting) are not possible, full-time caregiving must be considered. Providing a 24-hour contact telephone number and daily calls from a nurse or ancillary volunteer can give social support that might not be available from family members.

When family members can support and care for their relatives, nurses can provide information that will assist in preparation for modifications in home arrangements that will need to be made. "Families must adapt to additional sources of stress, decreased flexibility, restricted options, increased responsibilities, family separation/isolation, and probably an increased financial burden," noted Jassak (1992, p. 874). Even when family members are agreeable to caregiving, they may not always be able to perform the skills and assume the responsibilities that the patient with cancer requires. Providing choices and information on community services and available assistance can help to build a foundation for family decision making. As the illness progresses, this information will continue to be helpful if difficult decisions must be made.

From Independence to Dependence

The clinical manifestations of advancing cancer include pain, cachexia, and anorexia. Any or all of these symptoms will decrease a patient's ability to perform self-care. These symptoms often precede the need for palliative care. The shift from self-care to assisted care can be an emotional crisis for patients who have a high need for control.

Symbols for loss of physical control are associated with patterns of elimination. Bowel and bladder incontinence is degrading, especially for people who need to maintain total control over life events. Depression and expression of suicidal thoughts indicate psychological loss of control. Nurses must explore their patients' previous repertoire of coping strategies to identify interventions that will provide support.

Family Teaching

Hileman et al. (1992) identified very important caregiver needs that were not satisfied. These needs were called barrier needs. "The greatest barrier needs identified . . . were information about symptoms, the future, treatment side effects, and community resources" (p. 774). Major barrier needs were identified, in order of importance to the caregiver, as psychological needs, information needs, and patient-care needs.

Initial nursing interviews with caregivers can greatly reduce stress when questions about community resources, future expectations of needs for patients, and information about the underlying reasons for symptoms are provided. This information must be given verbally, but related written materials should be provided to caregivers for easy reference. When appropriate, referrals to outside support agencies may be beneficial to patients and caregivers. These agencies can include specific community services for support groups, homecare supply services, and a variety of other vendors.

Caregiving Tasks

As many members of the family as possible should be instructed in basic physical patient care. Children can be a source of assistance when they are given simple tasks to do, such as gathering items needed for personal care or dressing changes. They can provide company and can read books or newspapers to weakened elderly relatives.

Some caregivers must learn more complex skills when medical equipment is needed at the bedside. Nurses can assist by providing organizing materials, such as flow sheets, and specific written instructions directed toward individual patient needs. When manuals are confusing to caregivers, nurses must simplify the instructions and reinforce them with follow-up calls and visits.

Realistic Planning

The demands caused by elderly patients' needs vary greatly. Different forms of cancer can progress slowly, become stable, or progress rapidly after being stable for some time. Nurses must not lose sight of the pervasive nature of cancer and the effect on each family member. Some families will cancel plans indefinitely, while others will continue with planned activities, always knowing that a cancellation at the last minute may be necessary. This poses a unique challenge for homecare nurses. An astute, professional nurse must monitor each patient and family situation. Family teaching and support should be planned before families face crises in caregiving or decision making.

The Impact of Family Caregiving

Family caregiving requires that the personal and physical needs of each member are met regularly. Emotional needs must include ventilation of feelings and a break from continuous, intense, and stressful caregiving. Physical needs include adequate nutrition and sleep.

Nursing interventions that reduce feelings of anxiety, helplessness, and loss throughout the cancer experience must support patient and family caregiver needs. The cancer experience has been called an unending roller coaster of emotion. An upward ride does not last long enough for revitalization of the patient or family caregiver before another downward spin begins. The terminal phase is expectedly more demanding and emotionally draining on all people involved.

"Changes in the scope of responsibilities imposed by illness, repeated hospitalizations, and diminished occupational involvement mandate the reassessment of family roles and responsibilities" (Jassak, 1992, p. 872). Several issues related to family dynamics interact with the family response to a cancer diagnosis. Research has identified similarities among family members related to several issues associated with the cancer experience. Most show great concern related to advanced disease and the terminal stage.

During the illness progression, family members and caregivers may display a wide range of needs while taking on different roles. These roles can range from being a partner in care with the nurse to personally needing nursing interventions.

When caregivers are planning to be partners in care, nurses must assess the type of treatment plan being initiated and the caregivers' ability to perform the needed skills. Nurses should assess the caregiver's willingness to learn skills and identify potential problems, such as barriers to learning. Nurses should provide opportunities for return demonstration of newly learned skills. The plan should provide time for discussion and evaluation of the caregivers' ability to manage medications and treatments. Information on identification of side effects, adverse reactions, and toxic reactions to the medications must be included in the teaching plan. Nurses should provide written material for reference in all aspects of care required and provide time to review the information with patients and family caregivers throughout care.

Dealing With Family Caregiver Guilt

When communication problems have created conflict within the family for extended time periods, nurses will need to provide guidance to encourage assertive, instead of aggressive, expressions of feelings. Family members frequently engage in discussions of guilt over missed opportunities to be with the patient before this illness. Nurses need to provide time to support family members who need to let go of negative feelings over past events that cannot be changed. Providing guidance and an outlet for these feelings will strengthen communication and permit supportive activities between patients and other family members.

Physical Strain

Cancer-related fatigue is considered the number-one side effect of cancer treatments. As a patient's illness progresses and the ability for self-care diminishes, the caregiver may assume more physical care duties. When lifting and physical strength requirements become a normal part of everyday care, nurses may need to obtain adjuncts to home care. Lifting devices are beneficial in transferring patients from bed to chair and back; however, they take a large amount of space to store and use. Patients may need to be moved to larger rooms in the home. Often, dining rooms or living rooms are larger than bedrooms and are better suited for care modalities during the terminal stages of cancer care at home.

When only one caregiver is involved with home care, more frequent relief of the main caregiver will be needed to prevent exhaustion and frustration. Nurses can assist family members in arranging a schedule that will accommodate most family members' routines. When this is not possible, nurses can inform caregivers of alternative solutions, such as respite care.

Respite Care

When caregivers have other life events that require letting go of the caregiver role for a brief time or when exhaustion or emotional fatigue results from uninterrupted caregiving for long periods of time, temporary relief usually can be found. Respite care is a temporary substitute for family caregivers during terminal phases of cancer. Two common forms of respite care are informal neighbor/friend assistance and formal hospice facilities for patients with cancer. Some long-term care facilities offer hospice services in addition to the hospice unit in a hospital.

Informal assistance is very personal and well meaning. Short, frequent breaks in caregiving patterns with informal assistance are one way to involve these nonmedical helpers. Respite care offered through a church or community organization in which parish nursing or other trained hospice homecare volunteers are available is safe and effective. These organizations may even include homemaking services for several visits and other assistance for frazzled caregivers. When care becomes so intense that caregivers are in need of respite, professional assistance may be the best alternative. The care that is required may be too overwhelming for nonmedically trained people.

Formal hospice programs generally offer facilities for respite care of terminal patients with cancer. This inpatient care is usually provided for two to five days only. If longer respite is required, because of emerging circumstances, arrangements may need to be made with extended or long-term care facilities for additional time. The hospital setting is not an appropriate choice for terminal hospice patients unless procedures must be performed or medications for comfort must be regulated.

Family caregivers have stated that having a few hours or days of time away from the physical and emotional endurance needed to care for terminally ill family members provides an opportunity to let go of the intense stress and become energized for continued care. Hull (1992) identified this sentiment during interviews with families that had selected respite care.

Patients frequently appreciate respite programs because they reduce the guilt of requiring so much time and attention from caregivers. Some families do not use respite care because of a fear that a terminal patient will die while they are away. Other families use the hospice facility for the death event only because they are especially uncomfortable with their loved one dying at home. When the family plans to use the hospice facility, the transfer must be expedited during the final day or hours before the anticipated death event (Hull, 1992).

Patient Teaching and the Pain Experience

The dynamics of pain management must be understood for care of patients with terminal cancer pain. Nursing care for terminal cancer pain should include appropriate medication at intervals that preclude patients requesting medication for pain exacerbation. This should be accomplished while an acceptable level of alertness is maintained. Pain management should be aimed at control of both the physical and emotional aspects of the pain experience. Patients who are able to administer pain medication should be allowed to do so. Self-control of time and dosage of pain medicine reduces anxiety and stress associated with the fear of being in pain and not having medication available. Nurses must give patients instructions on maintaining a flow sheet for keeping records of all medication administered. The homecare nurse can make this flow sheet. The sheet should include the date, time, pain rating (e.g., scale of 1 to 10), specific medication and dosage, appropriate vital signs, level of arousal, and a comment section. See Chapter 9 for more information on pain management.

Pre- and Post-Chemotherapy Treatments

Before beginning outpatient treatment regimens of chemotherapeutic agents, family caregiver assessment and teaching are necessary. Assessment and instruction regarding maintaining a clean home environment, adequate plumbing, available telephone service, nutritional elements (e.g., refrigerator, stove, food supplies), and access to emergency assistance are essential. Caregivers must be able and willing to help with potentially changing physical conditions.

Post-treatment precautions vary according to the chemotherapy agents given. During the immediate 48 hours after most chemotherapy agents are administered, precautions related to blood, vomitus, and excreta need to be exercised. Caregivers should wear disposable surgical latex gloves and protective disposable gowns or aprons. Bed linens must be handled in the same manner as contaminated gloves and clothing. These items must be placed in impervious trash containers and disposed of according to local health department regulations. Nurses must always determine the agent and post-treatment recommendations prior to preparing a homecare plan.

Infection

The immunosuppressive effects of many types of chemotherapy create the potential for infection. Caregivers must be carefully instructed and monitored on handwashing techniques. The teaching plan should include handwashing before and after giving care and handling food, after toileting activities, and before any patient treatments.

Visitors may need to be restricted during the days following chemotherapy when the patient's immune system is depressed. An alternative may be to use facial filter masks; however, clear adherence to the proper use of the masks is essential. Exposure to anyone recently vaccinated with diphtheria, pertussis, and typhoid (DPT) or measles, mumps, and rubella (MMR) must be restricted. These vaccines carry a high risk of infection in immunosuppressed individuals.

Nausea and Vomiting

Caregivers have identified nausea and vomiting as the most distressing side effects of chemotherapy. These side effects may be acute, persistent, or delayed. Caregivers will need to be instructed in assessing and reporting the frequency, severity, duration, and pattern of symptoms following chemotherapy. Interventions should be planned and may include relaxation techniques, distraction, and guided imagery. Some caregivers are asked to administer antiemetic drugs up to an hour before therapy in an attempt to reduce or eliminate nausea and vomiting.

Nausea and vomiting can create an alteration in nutrition and result in a deficiency of body requirements. A dietary record of food intake, eating habits, and food and fluid preferences is recommended. Caregivers will need to be instructed to weigh patients regularly and keep records of intake and output. Teaching plans must include the rationale for keeping these observations and records. Research surveys of caregivers have identified a need for information related to the duties assigned to them by the homecare nurse. Compliance is higher when caregivers clearly understand rationales.

Stomatitis

A common post-treatment discomfort is stomatitis, an inflammation of the mucous membranes of the mouth. Stomatitis affects the oral cavity, causing difficulties with oral food intake, discomfort during tongue movement, infection, and bleeding. Saline mouth rinses have been identified as superior to hydrogen peroxide mixtures for the treatment of stomatitis (Coleman, 1995; Dose, 1995; Tombes & Gallucci, 1993). The most common formula for saline solution as a mouth rinse is to dissolve 1/2 teaspoon of table salt in eight ounces of water. When sodium bicarbonate rinse is preferred, the solution is made by mixing one teaspoon of sodium bicarbonate to one pint of warm water (Dose). Commercial mouthwashes have been demonstrated to dry and irritate oral tissues when used frequently (Dose).

Oral discomfort can be treated with clotrimazole troches. The high sucrose provides a somewhat sweet taste. Oral swishing and expectorating a topical anesthetic such as dyclonine hydrochloride 0.5%–1% solution is another way to decrease the oral discomfort of stomatitis (Dose, 1995).

Candida can be found in the mouth and esophagus of patients with stomatitis. Healthcare providers may order oral treatment with nystatin, and nurses will give instructions to the family (Schneider & Hogan, 1993). The oral suspension should be swished and then swallowed three to four times daily until the infection clears (Dose, 1995).

Prevention of stomatitis should be attempted prior to the beginning of radiation or chemotherapy treatments. This care should center around the following.
1. Establishing a pattern of good nutrition
2. Maintaining an intake of protein and vitamins B and C
3. Drinking two liters of fluids daily
4. Maintaining meticulous oral hygiene
    a. Brushing and flossing teeth after meals and at bedtime
    b. Regular dental care before, during, and after treatments

An oral assessment should include careful examination of the teeth, lips, palate, tongue, mucous membranes, and gingiva and notation of any mouth odor (Eilers, Bergen, & Petersen, 1988).

Alopecia

Hair loss can be upsetting to patients and family caregivers. Although most hair loss is temporary after a chemotherapy cycle, sufficient regrowth may take as long as six months. Resources for obtaining a wig, scarf, or hat (cap) should be provided before chemotherapy begins. Caregivers must also be instructed in scalp and hair care. The following information is recommended for inclusion in the teaching plan.
• Use only gentle shampoo.
• Avoid hair dryers and curling irons.
• Avoid hair color and permanent waves or straightening solutions.
• Protect the scalp from direct sunlight; wear a scarf or cap outdoors.

Hair may be cut short as the initial signs of hair loss occur. Preparing the patient for excessive hair loss during brushing or combing will allay some of the shock of seeing large patches of hair loss after grooming.

Anorexia

Anorexia may be related to the cancer or its treatment. A challenge for family caregivers is identifying foods that are palatable without causing nausea and vomiting. Fluids must be maintained to prevent dehydration. Commercial supplements that are high in calories and protein are available at supermarkets and drug stores. These drinks can provide temporary nutritional support until patients are able to eat without nausea and vomiting. Consultation with a dietitian may be helpful in determining ways to maintain nutritional status. Family caregivers should understand the signs and symptoms of dehydration and malnutrition, and they should be instructed to notify the healthcare provider if identified.

Cachexia

Cachexia means generalized weakness, malnutrition, and severe illness associated with terminal cancer (Anderson, 1998). According to Lueckenotte (1996), "Therapy for the cachectic state is rarely successful unless the underlying cancer is treated" (p. 356). To counteract the malnutrition, a high-carbohydrate, high-protein diet can provide the needed nutrition for maintenance and tissue repair. When cachexia leads to bedrest, additional muscle wasting will result, further debilitating the patient. Passive range of motion may be given by the caregivers several times a day to prevent muscle contractions when the weakened state continues. See Chapter 10 for additional information about symptom management.

Pre- and Post-Radiation Treatments

More than 60% of all patients with cancer receive radiation therapy. Treatments are given for primary, adjuvant, or palliative therapy. Types of radiation therapy include external and internal treatments. The purpose of the therapy and the type determine the care needed by the older adult undergoing radiation treatments (Petty, 1997).

Preparation for radiation therapy that will be given on consecutive days for several weeks must be included in nursing care plans. Clothing should be loose and disposable in case the skin marks stain the fabric. If a radioactive agent is used, special preparations for home management are included. Teaching caregivers about the preparation, process, and follow-up associated with radiation therapy will help to reduce stress caused by treatment. Instructions must be individualized to the area being treated.

Fatigue During and After Radiation

Fatigue is an expected side effect of radiation therapy. It can begin during the third or fourth week of treatment and can persist for a few weeks following the end of therapy. Some patients find that the fatigue is less noticeable on some days while more obvious on other days. Spacing activities with rest periods helps to provide the needed balance to prevent exhaustion. Reassuring the patient that the fatigue is not a sign that the cancer is spreading is important (Bender, Yasko, & Strohl, 1996).

Skin Care

Skin areas respond differently to the various types and lengths of radiation treatments. Some skin will have a mild erythema without discomfort, while other skin will look like a second-degree burn. This moist desquamation is not actually a burn but rather a skin reaction. Instruction should include keeping the treatment area dry until specific instructions are given that permit washing with a mild soap, rinsing well, and patting dry gently. Water should be warm or cool but never hot. The skin markings must not be removed until all treatments are completed. Powders, lotions, creams, alcohol-containing liquids, and deodorants should be avoided on the treatment areas. Skin care includes avoiding exposure to direct sunlight, chlorinated swimming pools, and temperature extremes (e.g., heating pads) (Black & Matassarin-Jacobs, 1997).

Site-Specific Reactions

Depending upon the treatment area, differing reactions are possible. When head and neck treatments are required, mucositis, xerostomia, and radiation caries can occur. If the throat is involved, esophagitis, dysphagia, nausea, and vomiting are not uncommon. Cystitis and urethritis can accompany treatments to the lower abdomen, while tenesmus can result from colon and rectal radiation therapy. Some people experience alopecia, while others have bone marrow suppression. Blood counts may be required weekly when bone marrow suppression is anticipated. Symptom management for the site-specific reactions is similar to that given for responses to chemotherapy (Petty, 1997).

Emotional Support

The fear of radiation treatments stems from myths that need to be addressed and discussed openly with the patient and caregivers. Some myths concern the fear of being radioactive and bringing harm to people nearby. It may be seen as a last resort after all else has failed or may be associated with expectations of severe side effects. These fears and misconceptions can be dispelled through providing the patient an opportunity to express feelings about receiving radiation treatments (Dunn-Daly, 1994).

Community and Home-Based Services

Hospice Care

Hull (1992) studied the benefits of palliative home care of patients with advanced cancer. In this study, family members were the primary caregivers for their dying relatives. Additionally, the family caregivers identified hospice services as invaluable in keeping patients at home until a peaceful death occurred. Services named were physical care, counseling services, volunteer assistance, respite care, support at the time of death, and bereavement follow-up. Most hospice programs will accept patient enrollment if a physician has determined that death is expected within a six-month period. Before that time determination, family caregiving can be supplemented by home health care.

Neither the patient nor family members may have considered hospice care. Nurses can provide patient and family teaching about home or inpatient supportive care offered by a hospice program. The goals of hospice care are appealing to most patients at a time when the disease process seems out of control. Patient and family teaching about hospice care should include information on stabilizing and controlling symptoms, especially pain, while providing respite services for primary caregivers as needed.

Home Healthcare Services

Patients, family members, and healthcare providers mutually select home healthcare services prior to hospital discharge. Although planning includes discharge teaching by the nurse, patients often do not understand the problems with a transition from the hospital to the home setting. Equipment support and immediate physical assistance may not be readily available at home. Every attempt should be made, prior to hospital discharge, to discuss potential problems that might occur in the home. If potential problems are environmental, temporary adjustments should be planned prior to discharge. Environmental adjustments could be modifications to the bathroom (elevated toilet or safety bars on the tub), doorways (widen for wheelchair), and inside communication systems (call bell or intercom). Preplanned homecomings can reduce the stress involved in the transition from hospital to home.

Two basic types of homecare services are available to patients in most areas. High technological home care usually refers to infusion therapy that may include hydration, antibiotic and/or antifungal IV therapy, blood administration, IV pain therapy, and total parenteral nutrition therapy. The second type of home care is the traditional homecare nursing service.

When a family, patient, or physician requests home healthcare services, an initial pre-illness lifestyle assessment is recommended. Areas to be assessed include patient and family patterns of problem solving used in the past, both as a whole and as individual family members. Emotional changes related to the diagnosis of cancer must be assessed, especially related to a history of depression. Changes in daily activity levels and performance ability are also important. Nurses must identify patients' perceptions of the present illness and its prognosis and also planned treatment modalities. Nurses should identify family members or friends who will be sources of social, emotional, and physical support during the cancer treatment or palliative care period.

An unhurried demeanor is crucial during nursing care visits. Permitting patients to express fears, negative and positive thoughts, and feelings can be helpful in reducing patient and caregiver anxiety. Nurses must recognize patients' overt or covert expressions or feelings of loss of control over life and health. They must motivate patients to live for each day and encourage families to discuss the experiences that they have known or participated in with the patient during previous years to help to maintain patient self-esteem.

Maintaining control over daily activities and life decisions is an important need for elderly patients with cancer. Encouraging patients and caregivers to learn all that is available regarding the established treatment plan can foster this control. Nurses can be a source of instruction regarding the plan of care and function as an effective referral agent for needs that are beyond the role of the home caregiver. Keeping patients and caregivers fully aware of any special needs, along with information on the referral plan, will promote a sense of control over an unfamiliar healthcare system. Referrals to psychosocial agencies or for other homecare services, such as dietary consults for preparation of special menus and alternative food preparation (e.g., liquefying or adding bulk), may need to be anticipated.

Complementary Modalities

Physical care management is just one part of the nursing care that homebound elderly patients with cancer need. Complementary self-care modalities can be especially helpful in this setting (Albright, 1997). The use of guided imagery, relaxation therapy, and progressive life review can be beneficial. According to Shealy (1996), "Relaxation therapy allows the mind-body complex to get on with its own healing work, restoring internal harmony and creating afresh the conditions for optimal functioning" (p. 116).

Acupuncture and acupressure are only recommended for reducing nausea in some people and easing pain. However, they are not recommended for use on damaged skin or where metastases have been noted. Hypnosis and self-hypnosis may be of some use as a method to alleviate pain and reinforce hope. Relaxation techniques have been helpful as a supportive therapy to ease muscle tension and reduce anxiety and feelings of despondency (Bettschart, Glaeske, Langbein, Saller, & Skalnik, 1998).

Ancillary Healthcare Services

Services can be provided to help family caregivers with some household and shopping chores. This is especially important for elderly spouse, sibling, or parent caregivers. Area Agencies on Aging are funded from a combination of federal grants, state aid, and local support. Homemaker and chore assistance can be obtained by contacting the local agency and applying for these services. A waiting list may be in place in some areas of the country; therefore, patients should seek information and apply for services before the services are actually needed.

Medication Needs

Pharmacotherapeutic services can be arranged with most pharmacies. Homecare nurses must be aware of patients' insurance plans and any limitations on pharmacy services. If health plans other than Medicare are selected, pharmacy services must be secured from approved lists of drug stores. Families must budget for the cost of drugs to be given at home if patients are on Medicare unless a supplemental insurance policy is available to cover prescription drugs.

Transportation Services

Elderly caregivers may not have automobiles available for trips to physicians' offices or outpatient clinics. Most major metropolitan areas offer ride services for the elderly in taxi cabs or service vans. These services may or may not be convenient for elderly caregivers and elderly patients. Times and routes often do not coincide with medical appointments, waiting times, and outpatient services that might be ordered during visits. Depending on the location of the pickup service, several additional passengers may need to be picked up before traveling to the site. Long rides can create difficulties for elderly patients who are ill. Any of these difficulties may discourage further use, even when an office visit is needed.

Some hospice organizations and regional healthcare centers provide transportation to their clinics and outpatient facilities. Nurses must become familiar with all of the possible transportation services that elderly homecare patients can use. Church members and the local cancer society may provide sources of transportation or ride services when chemotherapy and radiation treatments are needed.

Establishing a Legacy

A legacy is an important aspect of aging and of dying. Establishing a written or verbal record of life events can be an enriching and emotional experience. The process of writing or recording the life review as a legacy to future generations is usually a project of love within a family. Questions need to be developed that will provide insight into life at a time that may seem foreign to younger family members or nonfamily narrators. The legacy of a life review can take place over many sessions, with questions asked by different family members. The patient's ability to participate and continue with one or more sessions is a commitment that could quite possibly become too draining to finish.

Often the process promotes an acceptance of impending death. Acknowledging the reality of the situation may serve to foster resolution and acceptance of the terminal state. Mental health professionals, skilled in guided autobiographies, are helpful in guiding reminiscing during a review. Patients may resolve resentment and past hostility. A greater meaning may be achieved as a legacy is left for future generations (Birren & Deutchman, 1991).

Final Care and Death at Home

Anticipated death can be a long-term event for many family members. During the final weeks, emotional preparation can include bargaining for less or no pain for the loved one. Psychologically, many family members rehearse the impending death. The uncertainty of daily events can become a major stressor. Grief resolution is a highly variable component after the death of a loved one. Nurses must remember that no timetable exists for actual grief and bereavement experiences following an unexpected or anticipated death. Family follow-up support must be a part of nursing plans of care for elderly patients with cancer in the home setting.

When Death Occurs

Nurses need to recommend plans for final arrangements. Family members should be encouraged to discuss funeral and burial plans with patients or each other before the final days of life. Details can be delayed, but significant decisions are best made before the actual grief experience following the death. Hospice nurses often are called to be with families at the time of death to provide support and guidance in immediate activities that satisfy both health and legal authorities. A skilled hospice nurse is an invaluable asset to the family during and immediately following the death.

Follow-up care with family members is an important element of nursing care of the family. Contact with families on the day after the funeral, one week later, one month later, and six months later is appropriate hospice nursing follow-up. The contact can be by telephone during the first month and by mail in the following time periods.

Conclusion

As the number of elderly homecare patients with cancer continues to increase, nurses will be asked to provide nursing care, direction, support, and instructions on caregiving to patients and caregivers. Identifying the needs of home caregivers will continue to be a challenge in the changing environment of the healthcare delivery systems. This challenge will include having plans that provide for ever-changing needs over time. A significant element in preparing the patient, family, and home caregivers for needs following discharge from the hospital must include a strong plan for meeting the needs of psychological and informational support and also physical care. Community linkages might involve referral for initial counseling and obtaining informational literature and videotape programs on issues facing caregivers of elderly patients with cancer. Professional nursing involvement can be narrowly focused or broad-based depending on healthcare provider orders, family needs and preferences, and the nature of the course of illness. Consistent follow-up evaluation is essential to decide the effectiveness of the home-based care plan. Meeting the physical, psychological, and informational needs of patients and their family caregivers will demand all of the homecare nurse's skills.

References

Albright, P. (1997). *Complementary therapies.* Allentown, PA: People's Medical Society.

American Association of Retired Persons. (1998). *A profile of older Americans, 1998.* Washington, DC: Author.

Anderson, K.N. (Ed.). (1998). *Mosby's medical, nursing, and allied health dictionary.* St. Louis: Mosby.

Bender, C.M., Yasko, J.M., & Strohl, R.A. (1996). Cancer. In S.M. Lewis, I.C. Collier, & M.M. Heitkemper (Eds.), *Medical-surgical nursing: Assessment and management of clinical problems* (4th ed.) (p. 282). St. Louis: Mosby.

Bettschart, R., Glaeske, G., Langbein, K., Saller, R., & Skalnik, C. (1998). *The complete book of symptoms & treatments.* Boston: Element Books, Inc.

Birren, J.E., & Deutchman, D.E. (1991). *Guiding autobiography groups for older adults: Exploring the fabric of life.* Baltimore: Johns Hopkins University.

Black, J.M., & Matassarin-Jacobs, E. (1997). *Medical-surgical nursing. Clinical management for continuity of care* (5th ed). St. Louis: Mosby.

Chapman, K.J., & Pepler, C. (1998). Coping, hope, and anticipatory grief in family members in palliative home care. *Cancer Nursing, 21,* 226–234.

Coleman, S. (1995). An overview of the oral complications of adult patients with malignant hematological conditions who have undergone radiotherapy or chemotherapy. *Journal of Advanced Nursing, 22,* 1085–1091.

Corbin, J.M., & Strauss, A. (1988). *Unending work and care managing chronic illness at home.* San Francisco: Jossey-Bass.

Dose, A.M. (1995). The symptom experience of mucositis, stomatitis, and xerostomia. *Seminars in Oncology Nursing, 11,* 248–255.

Dunn-Daly, C.F. (1994). Nursing care and adverse reactions of external radiation therapy: A self-learning module. *Cancer Nursing, 17,* 236–256.

Eilers, J., Bergen, A.M., & Petersen, M. (1988). Development, testing, and application of the oral assessment guide. *Oncology Nursing Forum, 15,* 325–330.

Hileman, J.W., Lackey, N.R., & Hassanein, R.S. (1992). Identifying the needs of home caregivers of patients with cancer. *Oncology Nursing Forum, 19,* 771–777.

Hull, M.M. (1992). Coping strategies of family caregivers in hospice homecare. *Oncology Nursing Forum, 19,* 1179–1187.

Jassak, P.F. (1992). Families: An essential element in the care of the patient with cancer. *Oncology Nursing Forum, 19,* 871–876.

Landis, S.H., Murray, T., Bolden, S., & Wingo, P.A. (1998). Cancer statistics, 1998. *CA: A Cancer Journal for Clinicians, 48,* 15.

Lueckenotte, A.G. (1996). *Gerontologic nursing.* St. Louis: Mosby.

Otto, S.E. (1995). *Pocket guide to oncology nursing.* St. Louis: Mosby.

Petty, J. (1997). Treatment modalities for neoplastic disorders. In J.M. Black & E. Matassarin-Jacobs (Eds.), *Medical-surgical nursing. Clinical management for continuity of care* (5th ed.) (pp. 562–590). Philadelphia: Saunders.

Schneider, S.M., & Hogan, R. (1993). Cancer. In B. Long, W. Phipps, & V. Cassmeyer (Eds.), *Medical-surgical nursing: A nursing process approach* (3rd ed.) (pp. 182–227). St. Louis: Mosby.

Shealy, C.N. (1996). *Alternative medicine.* Rockport, MA: Element Publishers.

Tombes, M.B., & Gallucci, B. (1993). The effects of hydrogen peroxide rinses on the normal oral mucosa. *Nursing Research, 42,* 332–337.

Chapter Five

Nursing Care of the Older Adult With Lung Cancer

Ann Schmidt Luggen, PhD, RN, CS, CNAA, ARNP

Introduction

Lung and bronchial cancer are the greatest causes of cancer deaths in men and women in the United States. They are by far the greatest cause of morbidity and mortality in world cancer deaths. In the early 1900s, lung cancer was a medical oddity. Today, lung cancer is the leading cause of cancer deaths worldwide.

Epidemiology

The incidence of lung cancer is increasing in elderly men and women (Lindsey & Sarna, 1996). Sixty-one percent of cases are found in patients older than 65 years of age, and 36.7% of cases are in those 65–74. Two-thirds of all deaths from lung cancer are in those older than 65.

Incidence

The highest incidence of lung and bronchial cancer is in older adults. The number of estimated new cases of lung cancer in the United States for 1999 is 171,600—94,000 in men and 77,600 in women (Landis, Murray, Bolden, & Wingo, 1999). Of men ages 60–79, 1 in 15 will develop lung cancer. Of women ages 60–79, 1 in 25 will develop lung cancer, with a birth to death chance of 1 in 18.

Mortality

The estimated number of deaths from lung and bronchial cancer for 1999 is 158,900—90,900 in men and 68,000 in women. In men ages 60–79, 60,721 died in 1995 (Landis et al., 1999). In men 80 and older, nearly 15,000 died that year. The mortality rate of lung cancer in men began to decline in the late 1980s; however, it still kills more than twice as many men as prostate cancer, the second leading cancer cause of death in men. African American men have the highest mortality rates for lung cancer.

Lung cancer kills more women than any other cancer in the United States. Lung cancer has surpassed breast cancer as the leading cancer cause of death in women and will account for 25% of all female cancer deaths in 1999 (Landis et al., 1999). In 1995, 37,426 women ages 60–79 died of lung cancer. Of women 80 and older, 11,463 died that year.

By race and ethnicity, lung cancer kills 102 per 100,000 African American males, compared with 70 Caucasians, 40 American Indians, 35 Asian/Pacific Islanders, and 32 Hispanics (all per 100,000). In women, 33.6 Caucasian women die per 100,000 compared to 32.7 African Americans, 19.6 American Indians, 15 Asian/Pacific Islanders, and 11 Hispanics (all per 100,000) (American Cancer Society, 1999; Landis et al., 1999).

Survival

The five-year survival rate of people with lung cancer has changed minimally in the past 20 years. From 1974–1994, survival rates for Caucasians increased from 13% to 15%, remained unchanged in African Americans at 11%, and are between 12% and 14% in all races. Only pancreatic cancer has a lower survival rate according to world data (Landis et al., 1999). The United States has the highest survival rate for lung cancer in the world, with only an 8% survival rate in Europe and developing countries (Landis et al.).

Etiology

Tobacco

The risk of lung cancer in heavy smokers is 10–25 times greater than the risk in nonsmokers (Groenwald, Frogge, Goodman, & Yarbro, 1998). Smoking is responsible for 90% of lung cancers (Lind, 1998). Multiple factors determine risk and include
- Number of cigarettes smoked/day
- Duration of smoking (number of years)
- Age at which smoking began
- Inhalation pattern
- Tar content of cigarettes smoked.

Tobacco is classified as a complete carcinogen. A complete carcinogen contains initiator and promoter substances. Repeated exposure to promoter substances may cause malignant behavior at the cellular level, which may be repaired if promoters are withdrawn (Groenwald et al., 1998).

Passive tobacco smoke contains nearly all the carcinogens that are present in direct (active) smoke. Passive exposure accounts for approximately 30% of lung cancers (Groenwald et al., 1998).

Environmental and Occupational Exposure

Asbestos causes approximately 3%–4% of lung cancers and is synergistic with smoking in the development of cancer (Groenwald et al., 1998). Radon is an initiator and promoter and is also synergistic with cigarette smoke.

In industry, those people with significant exposure to copper, lead, zinc, gold, chromium, arsenic, nickel, coal, silica, hydrocarbons, chromethyl ether, vinyl chloride, and ionizing radiation are at higher risk for the development of lung cancer. Other possible factors include building materials, aerosol products, outside air contaminants, furs, cadmium, and beryllium (Groenwald et al., 1998).

Genetics and Carcinogen Exposure

The major risk factor for lung cancer is exposure to tobacco smoke. Other pollutants have also been identified as carcinogens with a propensity for lung tissue. Among these are heavy metals, asbestos, and radon. Many older adults have been exposed to heavy metals used in smelting and to asbestos through employment prior to the formation of Occupational Safety and Health Administration standards. These exposures greatly increase risks for lung cancer. In some areas of the country, older adults have been exposed to radon for decades. Radon is commonly found in tightly insulated houses built over naturally occurring radon gas.

According to Amos, Wu, and Spitz (1999), "only about 11% of tobacco smokers ultimately develop lung cancer, suggesting that genetic factors may influence the risk for lung cancer among those that are exposed to carcinogens" (p. 3). Differences in DNA repair mechanisms, cellular mitotic control, protease activity, immunocompetence, and metabolic enzymes may account for the reason that all cigarette smokers do not develop lung cancer (Iannuzzi & Toews, 1994). Research examining the DNA sequence of gene coding for the P-450 gene enzymes is being conducted. Inherited cancer genes seem to predispose some people to lung cancer (e.g., the relatives of patients with retinoblastoma have a 15-times greater risk of developing lung cancer) (Iannuzzi & Toews).

Poor DNA repair is independent of tobacco smoking and other carcinogen exposures. Previous research studies have shown that damaged components of DNA are not repaired sufficiently to prevent lung cancer in individuals with familial predisposition and exposure to carcinogens (Amos et al., 1999).

Pathology

Histology

Four histologic types account for 95% of all primary neoplasms of the lung (Iannuzzi & Toews, 1994). Seventy-five to 80% of lung cancers are classified as non-small cell lung cancer (NSCLC) (Sigmund, 1994). NSCLC is primarily identified as squamous cell carcinoma, adenocarcinoma, and anaplastic, large cell carcinoma. Survival in NSCLC is 16.8% in those 55–64 years of age and 12.9% in those age 65 and older (Lindsey & Sarna, 1996).

Twenty percent of lung cancers are small cell lung cancer (SCLC) (Iannuzzi & Toews, 1994). SCLCs are subclassified as oat cell carcinoma (90%) with intermediate and combined (mixed) making up the remaining 10% (oat cell carcinoma combined with adenocarcinoma or squamous cell carcinoma). Aggressive, rapidly growing neoplasms, SCLCs usually have metastasized at the time of diagnosis. The rate of survival for SCLC is 5.9% in those 55–64 years of age and 3.7% in those age 65 and older (Lindsey & Sarna, 1996) (see Table 5.1).

Table 5.1. Characteristics of Lung Cancers

Cancer Type	Frequency	Growth	Locus	Hormone Production	Optimum Therapy
Adenocarcinoma	25%	Variable	Peripheral	Rare	Surgery
Large cell	15%	Slow	Peripheral	Rare	Surgery
Squamous cell	35%	Slow	Hilar/Perihilar	Parathyroid hormone	Surgery
Small cell	25%	Rapid	Hilar/Perihilar	Multiple	Chemotherapy

Note. Based on information from Perry, 1994.

Cancer Sites

NSCLC: Squamous cell carcinoma is the most prevalent lung cancer cell type. It arises in the central bronchi in approximately 80% of patients and produces a cavitary lesion. Adenocarcinoma is linked to pulmonary fibrosis and generally occurs in areas of previous scarring in the periphery of the lung (Iannuzzi & Toews, 1994). Twenty-five percent of patients are asymptomatic at the time of diagnosis. Bronchoalveolar adenocarcinoma (5% of lung cancers) is an adenocarcinoma variant that spreads through the air spaces of the lungs and appears on the x-ray as multinodular lesions. It is the lung cancer least associated with tobacco smoking.

Anaplastic large cell carcinomas usually arise in the lung periphery and often are large and necrotic (Iannuzzi & Toews, 1994). Anaplastic large cell carcinoma is the least common of all lung cancers.

SCLC: Patients with small-cell lung cancer are seldom considered as surgical candidates. More than 90% of patients with SCLC are in stage III (locally advanced) or stage IV (systemic metastases) disease. Therefore, the Veteran's Administration Lung Cancer Study Group developed a system consisting of only two stages in 1973. These stages use only classifications of Limited Disease or Extensive Disease (Feld, Sagman, & LeBlanc, 1996).

Brain metastases are present in about 10% of patients with SCLC at the time of diagnosis. Median survival of 6–12 months is reported with current available therapy, but long-term disease-free survival is rare (Brown, Harken, Rabinovitch, Soriano, & Bunn, 1999).

Metastatic Disease Sites

Cancers of the lung are spread by direct extension, lymphatic invasion, and hematogenous routes. In NSCLC, metastasis usually occurs by direct extension or lymphatic invasion. Squamous cell carcinoma metastasizes late in the course of the disease. The routes of metastasis are the regional lymph nodes, the adrenal glands, and the liver. Adenocarcinoma metastasizes early in the disease process and frequently to bone (Iannuzzi & Toews, 1994).

Large cell anaplastic carcinoma is locally invasive and tends to metastasize widely early in the disease process and frequently is widespread, often to the gastrointestinal tract (Iannuzzi & Toews, 1994).

Clinical Presentation

Lung cancer may be present for many years prior to diagnosis. It occurs commonly in patients with chronic obstructive pulmonary disease (COPD), which may mask the signs and symptoms of cancer. The patient may exhibit systemic rather than specific symptoms (see Figure 5.1 and Table 5.2). Twenty-five to 30% of patients with NSCLC present with stage IV advanced disease (Parker, Tong, & Bolden, 1997).

Diagnosis and Staging

All patients should undergo a thorough health history, including a description of problems, past medical history, occupational history and exposure to potential carcinogens, family history, psychosocial history, review of all body systems, and examination of the pulmonary and lymphatic systems, including inspection, palpation, percussion, and auscultation. Diagnostic studies for lung cancer may include a chest x-ray with comparison to old x-rays to identify changes. The chest x-ray also may show enlargement of the hilum, a density with sharp or poorly defined borders, streaky infiltrates, signs of volume loss (atelectasis), a solitary nodule,

Figure 5.1. Systemic Symptoms

- Weakness
- Fatigue
- Anorexia
- Weight loss
- Anemia
- Cachexia
- Paraneoplastic syndromes (occur more commonly with small cell lung cancer)
- Cushing's syndrome
- Lambert-Eaton myasthenic syndrome
- Hypercalcemia
- Hypertrophic osteoarthropathy
- Neuromyopathies
- Syndrome of inappropriate secretion of antidiuretic hormone

cavitary lesion, peripheral mass, a mass larger than 3 cm, a mass with a doubling time of 1–18 months, eccentric calcifications, or pneumonia.

Computerized tomography (CT) of the chest will be performed to evaluate mediastinal lymph nodes, to confirm chest x-ray findings, and to locate hilar and mediastinal nodes. A CT scan of the area below the diaphragm will evaluate the liver, spleen, adrenal glands, and kidneys for metastatic disease. A CT scan is a noninvasive procedure requiring no anesthesia. The procedure is painless, but the patient must lie very still. IV contrast media may be used for better visualization. The patient may experience a warm sensation, flushing, bitter/salty taste, nausea or vomiting, and itching at insertion site. In rare cases, a severe allergic reaction to the contrast media may occur, possibly requiring cardiopulmonary resuscitation (Lind, 1998).

Magnetic resonance imaging may be ordered to visualize the perihilar and paravertebral lymph nodes. Once a lesion has been identified radiologically, a histologic diagnosis is needed. Several different techniques can be used to obtain a specimen to determine the tumor type.

Bronchoscopy is a fiberoptic visualization of the neoplasms and a way to obtain bronchial brushings and a biopsy for a histologic diagnosis.

Percutaneous needle biopsy is performed to obtain a histologic diagnosis for lesions not accessible by bronchoscopy, especially those lesions located in the lung periphery.

Mediastinoscopy allows direct visualization of the regional lymph nodes, and thoracoscopy is an examination of the pleural cavity, both of which are useful for diagnosis and staging of lung cancers.

Thoracentesis usually follows an x-ray finding of pleural fluid. Histologic diagnosis can be made using the pleural fluid obtained from this procedure (Iannuzzi & Toews, 1994). If pleural fluid is demonstrated on a chest x-ray, the fluid can be removed by thoracentesis. A large bore needle is inserted into the chest wall, and the fluid removed is sent for histologic analysis (Iannuzzi & Toews). Evaluation of sputum by cytology may provide a histologic diagnosis. Three consecutive sputum specimens must be submitted before a diagnosis is made.

A thoracotomy uses a surgical incision to obtain tissue samples as a biopsy (Iannuzzi & Toews, 1994). If palpable supraclavicular lymph nodes are present, a biopsy can be obtained to establish a histologic diagnosis.

Table 5.2. Tumor Presentations

Local Tumor Presentation	Regional Presentation	Distant Metastasis
Cough	Chest pain	Bone pain
Dyspnea	Hoarseness	Headache
Hemoptysis	Dysphagia	Abdominal pain
Wheezing	Superior vena cava syndrome	Lymphadenopathy
Pneumonia	Pancoast syndrome	Hepatomegaly
Fever	Horner's syndrome	Pleural effusion

Staging

The approach to staging lung cancer depends on the cell type, extent of tumor, nodal involvement, and metastases and guides the clinician in assessing prognosis and planning treatment. The tumor, nodes, and metastases (TNM) system is used to stage lung cancer (American Joint Committee on Cancer [AJCC], 1992). The AJCC, in conjunction with the International Union Against Cancer, developed the International Staging System. Each increase in T, N, or M correlates with an increasingly higher stage and a worsening prognosis (see Figures 5.2 and 5.3).

Prognosis

Performance status is the single most important determinant of prognosis (Perry, 1994). Those with Zubrod scores of 0, 1, or 2 or Karnofsky scores of 70% or greater survive longer than nonambulatory patients.

Patients with advanced NSCLC and 10% weight loss have a poor prognosis (Perry, 1994). In SCLC, poor prognosis is related to advanced stage, male sex, advanced age, elevated serum lactic dehydrogenase, elevated serum alkaline phosphatase, and decreased sodium.

Perry (1994) found operative mortality to be 6.2% with pneumonectomy, 2.9% with lobectomy, and 1.4% with segmentectomy or other small resection. Older adults, in one review, had higher mortality rates.

Older adults have local disease more often than do younger adults (Perry, 1994). This indicates a distinct histologic difference or behavior of neoplasms in older adults. Fewer older adults have SCLC, and they do have a higher incidence of squamous cell carcinoma and adenocarcinoma compared with younger adults. This suggests an increased likelihood of resectable and potentially curable cancer of the lung in older adults (Perry).

General Nursing Care

- Monitor patient and family response to possible diagnosis of lung cancer and related therapy (Pratt, 1998) .
- Perform a thorough pain assessment documenting areas of pain, areas of discomfort, and degree of pain.
- Discuss pain management techniques, if present, with emphasis on the need to stop pain before it becomes too painful (see Chapter 9).
- Identify baseline weight.
- Obtain diet history, food preferences, and dislikes.
- Perform a careful review of systems and physical examination.

Figure 5.2. Primary Tumor (T or PT), Regional Lymph Nodes (N), Distant Metastasis (M) (TNM) Staging System

Primary Tumor and Clinical Stage

T_x Presence of tumor proved but not visualized by x-ray or bronchoscopy

T_0 No evidence of primary tumor

Tis   Carcinoma in situ

T_1 Tumor 3 cm or less in diameter surrounded by lung or visceral pleura with no evidence of invasion proximal to lobar bronchus at bronchoscopy

T_2 Tumor more than 3 cm in diameter or any size tumor invading visceral pleura or presence of associated atelectasis or obstructive pneumonitis in hilar region but not the whole lung

T_3 Tumor of any size with direct extension into adjacent structure such as chest wall, diaphragm, or mediastinum; or tumor seen bronchoscopically to involve main bronchus less than 2 cm to the carina; or any tumor associated with atelectasis, obstructive pneumonitis of entire lung, or pleural effusion

T_4 Tumor of any size with invasion of mediastinum, cardiac involvement, invasion of great vessels, trachea, esophagus, vertebral body, or carina, or presence of malignant pleural effusion

Regional Lymph Nodes (N)

N_0 No demonstrable metastasis to regional lymph nodes

N_1 Metastasis to nodes in peribronchial or ipsilateral hilar region

N_2 Metastasis to ipsilateral lymph nodes within the mediastinum

N_3 Metastasis to contralateral mediastinal or hilar lymph nodes or contralateral or ipsilateral scalene or supraclavicular nodes

Distant Metastasis (M)

M_0 No distant metastases

M_1 Distant metastases to scalene or contralateral hilar lymph nodes, brain bone, liver, or lung

Figure 5.3. Tumor Staging

Stage 0:	Stage I:	Stage II:	Stage IIIa:	Stage IIIb:	Stage IV:
Tis $N_0 M_0$	$T_1 N_0 M_0$ $T_2 N_0 M_0$	$T_1 N_1 M_0$ $T_2 N_1 M_0$	$T_3 N_0 M_0$ $T_3 N_1 M_0$ $T_{1-3} N_2 M_0$	Any T $N_3 M_0$ T_4 Any N M_0	Any T Any N M_1

- If the patient has had a bronchoscopy under local anesthetic, evaluate for the return of the gag reflex after the procedure. Maintain the patient in a flat or semi-Fowler's position. Apply ice collar for 24 hours to decrease edema related to hyperextension of neck, then apply heat to reduce discomfort. Throat lozenges can be used for relief of discomfort when gag reflex returns. Observe the patient for laryngeal edema and laryngospasm. Apply oxygen and administer bronchodilators as ordered. Observe patient for bleeding and report any abnormalities to the physician. Pneumothorax is a possible complication of bronchoscopy. Evaluate the patient for diminished breath sounds, dyspnea, and cyanosis (Lind, 1998).

- Mediastinoscopy is performed under general anesthetic; therefore, the patient is allowed nothing by mouth before and after the procedure. Evaluate the patient for possible pneumothorax and report dyspnea, diminished breath sounds, and cyanosis. Administer oxygen and analgesics as ordered. Check the patient for evidence of bleeding and mediastinitis. Report a temperature elevation or cough to physician (Lind, 1998).

Nursing Diagnoses and Plan of Care

Primary nursing diagnoses related to lung cancer are listed below. Following identification of the diagnosis, nursing interventions are listed. Emotional support applies to all nursing interventions associated with older adults with cancer; therefore, it is not included with more specific actions.

Nursing diagnosis: Knowledge deficit related to a new medical condition, new treatments, surgical procedures (preoperative and postoperative), and medications

Supporting data: Verbalizes a deficiency in knowledge or skill/requests information; expresses an inaccurate perception of health status; unable to incorporate treatment plan into activities of daily living

Interventions:

- Educate patient/family regarding scheduled procedures and treatments.
- Discuss reasons for and measures to deal with side effects of treatments.
- Explain measures to limit activities as needed during treatment phases to conserve energy.
- Discuss measures to obtain adequate oxygenation.

Nursing diagnosis: Impaired gas exchange (actual or potential) related to decreased passage of gases between the alveoli of the lungs and the vascular system

Supporting data: Dyspnea on exertion; lethargy and fatigue; assumes a three-point position (sitting, bending forward with hands on knees); changes in respiratory rate or pattern

Interventions:

- Instruct patient/family in proper position and methods for air exchange.
- Maintain adequate humidity of inspired air.
- Instruct in safe use of oxygen in the home setting.

Nursing diagnosis: Fatigue related to treatment and treatment sequela

Supporting data: Verbalizes an overwhelming lack of energy; inability to perform usual activities of daily living; lethargy or listlessness

Interventions:

- Allow expression of feelings regarding the effects of fatigue on lifestyle.
- Determine fatigue level variations for daily activities using the Rhoten (1982) fatigue scale (0 = not tired, peppy; 10 = total exhaustion).
- Assist in planning tasks during periods of higher energy.
- Teach energy-conservation techniques (reduce trips up and down stairs, organize work items within easy reach, etc.).

Nursing diagnosis: Grief (actual or anticipatory) related to unknown prognosis of disease

Supporting data: Feelings of loss associated with thoughts of terminal illness; potential loss of body image when surgery may be recommended

Interventions:

- Support the patient's/family's grief reactions.
- Recognize and reinforce strengths and weaknesses of coping skills.
- Identify agencies that provide ongoing support for patient/family.
- Assess patient/family for pathological grief reactions and refer as needed.

Treatment

Nearly half of patients with NSCLC have surgically unresectable disease at the time of presentation. Approximately one-third have resectable cancer (Sigmund, 1994) that is stage I B IIIa (Dunphy, 1999). Small cell lung cancers are not considered to be surgically treatable except in rare cases. In fact, TNM staging has not been found to be therapeutically or prognostically valuable and is not used (Sigmund). Chemotherapy is the treatment of choice (Dunphy).

Treatment decisions may be based on the patient's life expectancy and the presence of comorbid conditions (Duthrie & Katz, 1998). Age is not considered a contraindication to surgical resection, chemotherapy, or radiotherapy protocols.

Surgery is the preferred treatment and is considered curative in a small group of patients with NSCLC without metastases. Lobectomy (removal of a lobe of the lung) or pneumonectomy (removal of an entire lung) are procedures for removal of the primary tumor that is centrally located. Wedge resections are the most conservative approach and are used for small peripheral nodules or in those patients whose physical condition does not permit more extensive surgery (Groenwald et al., 1998). The survival rate for $T_1N_0M_0$ after resection is 80%–85% (Martini, 1993), 65% for $T_2N_0M_0$, and 72% overall for patients with stage I disease.

Prior history of cardiac disease, as commonly seen in older adults, doubles the risk of major operative morbidity (20% versus 10%) (Iannuzzi & Toews, 1994). However, in general, surgery in older adults has similar outcomes as surgery in younger adults (Burke & Walsh, 1998). Compromised pulmonary status from COPD may prohibit any surgical intervention and is contraindicated if evidence of extra-pulmonary metastases, scalene node metastases, metastases to the other lung, or inadequate pulmonary function exists (Lind, 1998).

Adjuvant Therapy

Radiotherapy

Radiation therapy is used more in elderly patients with lung cancer who have localized disease compared to younger patients (30% versus 14%) (Hillner et al., 1998). However, the therapy is used less often in elderly patients with distant metastases (55% versus 76%) (Hillner et al.). The disease is rarely curative, with only a small percentage surviving five years; however, complete regression occurs in approximately half of treated patients but with increasing incidence of local recurrence (Lindsey & Sarna, 1996).

External-beam radiotherapy is used alone with curative intent for stage I or II NSCLC when lung function is impaired or other conditions preclude surgery (Lind, 1998). A dose of 5,500–6,000 cGy is delivered to the midplane of the tumor.

The effects of radiotherapy on normal tissues, skin, and mucous membranes of older adults may be more pronounced (Burke & Walsh, 1998). Fatigue also can be a more pronounced problem in this patient population.

Preoperative or postoperative radiotherapy can be used as an adjuvant to surgery (Lind, 1998). Radiotherapy also is used for prophylaxis in patients with brain metastases and SCLC, but its value is unclear.

Chemotherapy

Chemotherapy is the treatment of choice for SCLC. It improves survival time to 12–18 months versus approximately 2 months without chemotherapy (Lind, 1998). Response rates of 80% have been reported (Perry, 1994). Chemotherapy also may be used for stage IIIa and IIIb NSCLS as an adjuvant to surgery (Lindsay & Sarna, 1996). However, NSCLC is relatively insensitive to chemotherapy, with responses of 25%–40% (Perry). Current chemotherapy regimens used in combination with radiotherapy or immunotherapy include the following.

- Cisplatin as a single agent is one of the most effective drugs against NSCLC. Cisplatin has a moderate antitumor effect but limited effect on survival (Parker et al., 1997).
- Etoposide and cisplatin or a carboplatin combination shows little increase in survival (Parker et al.).
- Topotecan exhibits modest activity against NSCLC (Perez-Soler, 1997).
- Cyclophosphamide + doxorubicin + vincristine
- Cyclophosphamide + doxorubicin + etoposide
- Paclitaxel
- Isotretinoin + interferon
- Ifosfamide + carboplatin + etoposide
- Cisplatin + mitomycin + vinblastine
- Vinorelbine + cisplatin
- Carboxyamidotriazole + paclitaxel

The chemotherapy agents listed above are only a partial list of combinations that are used in the treatment of NSCLC. Because of the rapid findings in research and the slower ability to disseminate findings, current periodicals can provide the most up-to-date information on chemotherapeutic agents and combinations.

Prior to 1990, six agents were used for the treatment of NSCLC: cisplatin, ifosfamide, mitomycin, vindesine, vinblastine, and etoposide. More recent additions to the therapy regimen are taxanes, camptothecin analogs, antimetabolites (gem), and new vinca alkaloids (vinorelbine), all of which show promise (Parker et al., 1997).

Combination therapies have not been well studied in older adults. Clinical trials are needed (Burke & Walsh, 1998). Toxicity in older adults is not well established. Clinicians should consider the normal changes that occur with aging and compare them with the toxicities of specific chemotherapeutic agents to anticipate problems. Such changes include the following (Engelking, 1996).

- Decreased absorption
- Decreased motility
- Decreased visceral blood flow
- Decreased active transport
- Increased pH and decreased acid production
- Decreased liver size, circulation, and enzyme activity
- Age-altered plasma proteins
  - Decreased serum albumin
  - Decreased bioavailability of protein-bound drugs
- Decreased biotransformation of drugs to active form: decreased formation of active metabolites, decreased inactivation of drug, and decreased drug clearance

Drug toxicities to consider in the elderly include the following.

- Cisplatin—Decrease dose 25%–50% with hepatic or renal compromise. Side effects include nausea and vomiting, nephrotoxicity, and ototoxicity (Engelking, 1996).
- Etoposide—Decrease dose 25%–50% with renal or hepatic clearance impairment. Drug causes bone marrow depression (Pratt, 1998). (Elderly have a diminished hematopoietic reserve.)
- Vinca alkaloids—Dose should be reduced for significant liver disease. May cause peripheral neuropathy, bone marrow depression, and ototoxicity.
- Paclitaxel—Causes paralytic ileus, bradyarrhythmias, and peripheral neurotoxicities.
- Ifosfamide—Delayed hepatic clearance (Engelking, 1996).

Treatment-Related Complications and Interventions

General Nursing Interventions

- Provide support and encourage the use of support groups or individual psychotherapy in dealing with cancer experience (Pratt, 1998). Older adults may have diminished social networks, which can result in social isolation (Luggen & Rini, 1995).
- Teach patients and families about risk factors and encourage smoking cessation (Pratt, 1998).
- Review medications and side effects. Compliance with medications is an issue in 25%–59% of patients (Engelking, 1996).
- Good symptom management is imperative for maintaining quality of life (see Chapter 11).
- Assist in evaluating reimbursement for medical/surgical care of older adults.

Surgery

Complications (Schmidt & Shell, 1994):

- Pneumonia occurs in 20%–40% of elderly postoperative patients (Pratt, 1998).
- Myocardial infarction and congestive failure are possible after surgery.
- Confusion following surgery is common in older adults. Look for causes (Pratt, 1998), such as
  - Sepsis
  - Alcohol withdrawal
  - Fluid and electrolyte imbalance
  - Hypoxia
  - Medications
- Fever
- Bleeding
- Cardiac arrhythmias, congestive heart failure, and fluid overload
- Airway obstruction, dyspnea, hypoxemia, and respiratory failure
- Pneumothorax
- Pulmonary embolus
- Prolonged hospitalization
- ICU psychosis
- Death

Interventions:

- Provide preoperative preparation for patients who will be on mechanical ventilation after lung surgery.
- Teach coughing and deep breathing.
- Splint incisions.
- Administer pain medication.
- Position patient to facilitate lung expansion.

Radiation

Side effects and complications:

- Immune status may be compromised further in an elderly patient with an already compromised immune system; infection may be a problem.
- Fatigue is a common side effect of radiation therapy. In older adults with lung cancer, fatigue often is already a serious problem that compromises activities and quality of life.

- Fibrosis of lung tissue often occurs some months after treatment has been completed, further compromising pulmonary status.
- Changes in skin and tissues
- Cases of esophagitis and dysphagia should be monitored.
- A new dry cough and fever may indicate pneumonitis from radiation.
- Pericarditis may occur; assess for chest pain, electrocardiogram changes, and pericardial friction rub (Groenwald et al., 1998).
- Erythematous skin reaction may occur up to three weeks post-therapy. The skin may peel, darken, or shed. Skin permanently thins and is more sensitive to damage.
- Late effects of radiation to the lung include narrowing of heart blood vessels (Pratt, 1998) (see Chapter 10).

Chemotherapy

Side effects and complications:
- Stomatotoxicity
- Delayed nausea and vomiting
- Diarrhea
- Cardiotoxicity (Pratt, 1998)
- Pulmonary toxicity (Pratt, 1998)
- Peripheral neuropathy (Pratt, 1998)
  Interventions:
- Teach patients about the side effects of chemotherapy.
- Teach patients how to manage side effects (see Chapter 10).
- Maintain good hydration, which is more of a problem in older adults.
- Follow laboratory data for monitoring chemotherapy toxicity.

Tumor-Related Complications and Interventions

Pleural Effusion (Schmidt & Shell, 1994)

- Lung cancer is one of the most common causes of pleural effusion.
- Twelve percent of patients with lung cancer present with pleural effusion.
- Impaired lung expansion occurs with poor gas exchange. Respiratory embarrassment, atelectasis, and recurrent infections are possible.
- Treat with repeated thoracenteses, pleurectomy, or intrapleural instillation of chemotherapy, intracavitary radioactive colloids, or a sclerosing agent such as an antibiotic.
- Sclerosing may be painful if tetracycline is used. Bleomycin is a sclerosing agent with little to no painful effect. Morphine is given prior to sclerosing.
- Malignant pleural effusion carries a poor prognosis; the goal is symptom control.
- Chest tube placement and interventions (Schmidt & Shell, 1994)
  - Will be used in patients receiving sclerosing therapies
  - May be used postoperatively
  - May be inserted to drain air or fluid
  - Will be sutured in place
  - Will be under sterile fluid (when suction pleural effusion is evident)
  - Usually will be clamped with pneumonectomy to allow filling of the thoracic cavity to prevent mediastinal shift (Lindsey & Sarna, 1996).

- Clamping a chest tube (suspicion of a leak) should be performed with *great caution.* If air or fluid cannot escape the pleural space but still is entering the space, a tension pneumothorax will occur with possible mediastinal shift and impaired blood flow to the heart.
- Examine sutures at chest tube site for redness, swelling, leakage, and purulence.
- Administer pain medications prior to procedures
- Maintain gravity for chest tube drainage; milking and stripping the tube should not be necessary unless tube is obstructed with clot.
- Administer a cough suppressant for dry cough but not for productive cough.
- Narcotics may be used for cough suppression; administer warm, humidified air.
- Avoid cigarette smoke (Groenwald et al., 1998).

Hemoptysis

- Patient with mild hemoptysis, less than 50 ml/24 hours, is treated as an outpatient.
- Patient with bleeding greater than 200 ml/24 hours requires immediate attention, hospitalization, and careful monitoring.
- Patient with hemoptysis should be positioned with lung in dependent position (Groenwald et al., 1998).

Dyspnea

- Assess patterns of occurrence, worsening, and best times.
- Plan coping strategies to conserve energy and minimize fatigue (Groenwald et al., 1998).
- Obtain blood gases.
- Assess breath sounds and document.
- Avoid deep suctioning.
- Assess dyspnea on a scale of 0–10 (0 = no dyspnea; 10 = intolerable dyspnea) and record results (Glover, 1995).
- Relieve dyspnea by using hydrocodone and morphine to reduce anxiety and ventilatory drive (Glover, 1995).
- Position patient in upright, leaning-forward position.
- Administer oxygen at appropriate amount of flow.
- Encourage pursed-lip breathing (Glover, 1995).

Pain (see Chapter 9)

Psychosocial Issues

- Explore with the patient and family any fears or financial concerns.
- Consult social service department for assistance.
- Evaluate need for skilled nursing placement.

Skin Irritation

- Use mild soap, warm water, and gentle patting to dry.
- Do not use hot packs, cold packs, creams, lotions, or powders if patient is receiving radiation therapy.
- Cornstarch may be used for pruritus.
- Encourage patient to change position frequently.

Anorexia and Weight Loss

- Provide a high-protein diet.

- Encourage frequent snacks.
- Encourage family to eat together as a social occasion.
- Provide soft, nonacidic foods if stomatitis or dysphagia is present.
- Increase calories and protein.
- Use meat base with soups and stews.
- Incorporate cottage cheese, fish, and other protein foods into diet.
- Use total parenteral nutrition as necessary as an adjunct to an oral diet.
- Promote wound healing and decrease the incidence of infection with a good nutritional status.

Additional Nursing Diagnoses

- Knowledge deficit related to the following.
  - A higher rate of functional illiteracy in those older than 65 years of age
  - Age-related sensory diminution
  - Misconceptions/fear related to cancer
  - Decreased social networks
  - Absence of teaching materials for older adults
  - Formal education of eighth grade or less (Engelking, 1996)
- Ineffective airway clearance
- Anxiety
- Activity intolerance
- Altered oral mucous membranes
- Potential for infection
- Altered nutrition—less than body requirements
- Body image disturbances
  - Sexual dysfunction
  - Impaired skin integrity
  - Nausea and vomiting (see Chapter 10 for a discussion of symptom management)

Palliation

Radiation therapy may be useful for control of symptoms such as severe cough, hemoptysis, pain, obstructive pneumonitis, and superior vena cava syndrome and for prolonging functional life of the person (Lind, 1998). Radiation also may decrease bone pain and has been used prophylactically for central nervous system involvement (Schmidt & Shell, 1994).

Laser therapy may be used for palliative treatment of endobronchial lesions (Schmidt & Shell, 1994). The therapy is less successful in treatment of smaller airway obstruction. Laser therapy can be performed on an outpatient basis and has a success rate of 75% with advanced lung cancer.

Chemotherapy may be given for palliation. The treatment is useful for managing symptoms such as superior vena cava obstruction.

Suffering occurs frequently in patients with lung cancer. In one study, 10% of patients reported no suffering and 50% reported a lot of suffering. The source of suffering is disability, pain, anxiety, change in daily activities, weakness, fatigue, and change in signs and symptoms (Lindsey & Sarna, 1996).

Depression is also a significant problem for many older adults. Depression can be alleviated in some cases with antidepressants. Spending time with the patient and assisting with a life review may be helpful in advanced stages of lung cancer (see Chapter 4).

Definitions

- Pancoast tumor: A tumor that occurs at the apex of the lung and extends to the thoracic outlet. The tumor can invade the sympathetic channels and stellate ganglion, causing Horner's syndrome. A Pancoast tumor is treated with preoperative radiation and an en bloc resection of the upper lobe of the lung and involved ribs. Pancoast syndrome consists of shoulder and arm pain and paresthesias of the C-7 or T-1 dermatome. The pain may radiate down the shoulder and arm (Faber, 1991).
- Horner's syndrome: Ipsilateral sweating of the face, ptosis of the eyelid, and a constricted pupil (Faber, 1991).
- Superior vena cava (SVC) obstruction: Edema of face, neck, and upper torso. Nipples may appear enlarged and swollen. Collateral venous circulation develops to the neck and upper body, and the patient displays an increased jugular venous pressure. SVC obstruction is secondary to peritracheal lymphadenopathy with compression of the great veins draining the head and upper trunk. SVC obstruction is seen most often in SCLC and right lung tumors (Lindsey & Sarna, 1996). Symptoms are severe coughing, blackouts with rising or bending, dyspnea, dysphagia, and periorbital edema. SVC obstruction requires emergency treatment with diuretics, dexamethasone, irradiation, and chemotherapy.
- Clubbing: Occurs in approximately one-third of cases, especially with squamous cell carcinoma. Classic clubbing appearance of fingers is characteristic and is caused by periosteal proliferation of long bones with increased blood flow to the affected extremity. Excision of the tumor causes dramatic relief. Clubbing occurs with hypertrophic pulmonary osteoarthropathy (HPO) (Faber, 1991).
- HPO: Osteitis occurring especially with squamous cell carcinoma. Most commonly occurs in radius, ulna, tibia, and fibula, with the patient developing swelling, erythema, and tenderness (Faber, 1991).
- Hypercalcemia: Usually associated with squamous cell carcinoma, which secretes parathyroid hormone-like polypeptide. It often is caused by metastases to the bone (Faber, 1991).
- Eaton-Lambert syndrome: Characterized by weakness of muscles, especially pelvic and thigh muscles. Electromyograph studies differentiate from myasthenia gravis (Faber, 1991).

Conclusion

Lung cancer is the leading cause of cancer-related deaths in North America and Europe. Nurses and related healthcare providers must be able to meet the needs of patients and families when this disease occurs. Recognizing the diagnostic features, common treatment modalities, and anticipated nursing interventions can provide the older adult with lung cancer with the means to maintain self-care for as long as possible.

References

American Cancer Society. (1999). *Cancer facts and figures—1999*. Atlanta: Author.
American Joint Committee on Cancer. (1992). *Manual for staging of cancer* (4th ed.). Philadelphia: Lippincott-Raven.

Amos, C.I., Wu, X., & Spitz, M.R. (1999). Is there a genetic basis for lung cancer susceptibility? In H.J. Senn, A., Costa, & V.C. Jordan, V.C. (Eds.), *Chemoprevention of cancer: A clinical update* (pp. 3–12). New York: Springer.

Brown, J., Harken, A.H., Rabinovitch, R., Soriano, A.F., & Bunn, P.A. (1999). Lung cancer. In M.H. Torosian (Ed.), *Integrated cancer management: Surgery, medical oncology, and radiation oncology* (pp. 443–476). New York: Marcel Dekker, Inc.

Burke, M., & Walsh, M. (1998). *Gerontologic nursing: Wholistic care* (2nd ed.). St. Louis: Mosby.

Dunphy, L.M.H. (1999). *Management guidelines for adult nurse practitioners*. Philadelphia: F.A. Davis.

Duthrie, E., & Katz, P.R. (1998). *Practice of geriatrics* (3rd ed.). Philadelphia: Saunders.

Engelking, C. (1996). Chemotherapy in the elderly. In M.B. Burke, G.M. Wilkes, & K. Ingwersen (Eds.), *Cancer chemotherapy* (2nd ed.) (pp. 519–534). Boston: Jones and Bartlett.

Faber, E.P. (1991). Lung cancer. In A.I. Holleb, D.J. Fink, & G.P. Murphy (Eds.), *American Cancer Society textbook of clinical oncology* (pp. 194–212). Atlanta: American Cancer Society.

Feld, R., Sagman, U., & LeBlanc, M. (1996). Staging and prognostic factors: Small cell lung cancer. In H.I. Pass, J.B. Mitchell, D.H. Johnson, & A.T. Turrisi (Eds.), *Lung cancer: Principles and practice* (pp. 495–509). Philadelphia: Lippincott-Raven.

Glover, J. (1995). Lung cancer. In C. Miaskowski (Ed.), *Oncology nursing* (pp. 111–123). New York: Delmar.

Groenwald, S.L., Frogge, M.H.., Goodman, M., & Yarbro, C.H. (1998). *Comprehensive cancer nursing review* (4th ed.). Boston: Jones and Bartlett.

Hillner, B.E., McDonald, M.K., Desch, C.E., Smith, T.J., Penberthy, L.T., & Retchin, S.M. (1998). A comparison of patterns of care of non-small cell lung carcinoma patients in a younger and Medigap commercially insured cohort. *Cancer, 83,* 1930–1937.

Iannuzzi, M.C., & Toews, G.B. (1994). Neoplasms of the lung. In J.H. Stein (Ed.), *Internal medicine* (4th ed.) (pp. 1733–1741). St. Louis: Mosby.

Landis, S., Murray, T., Bolden, S., & Wingo, P. (1999). Cancer statistics, 1999. *CA: A Cancer Journal for Clinicians, 49,* 8–31.

Lind, J. (1998). Nursing care of the client with lung cancer. In J. Itano & K. Taoka (Eds.), *Core curriculum for oncology nursing* (pp. 4448–4458). Philadelphia: Saunders.

Lindsey, A.M., & Sarna, L. (1996). Lung cancer. In R.M. McCorkle, M. Grant, M. Frank-Stromborg, & S.B. Baird (Eds.), *Cancer nursing: A comprehensive textbook* (2nd ed.) (pp. 611–634). Philadelphia: Saunders.

Luggen, A., & Rini, A. (1995). Assessment of social networks and isolation in community-based elderly men and women. *Geriatric Nursing, 16,* 179–183.

Martini, N. (1993). Operable lung cancer. *CA: A Cancer Journal for Clinicians, 43,* 201–214.

Parker, S.L., Tong, T., & Bolden, S. (1997). Cancer statistics. *CA: A Cancer Journal for Clinicians, 47,* 5–27.

Perez-Soler, R. (1997). Topotecan in the treatment of lung cancer and other solid tumors. *Seminars in Oncology, 24,* 520–534.

Perry, M.C. (1994). Lung cancer. In W. Hazzard, E. Bierman, & J. Blass (Eds.), *Principles of geriatric medicine and gerontology* (3rd ed.) (pp. 607–612). St. Louis: McGraw-Hill.

Pratt, P. (1998). Cancer considerations in the elderly. In A.S. Luggen, S. Travis, & S. Meiner (Eds.), *NGNA core curriculum for gerontological advanced practice nurses* (pp. 447– 467). Thousand Oaks, CA: Sage.

Rhoten, D. (1982). Fatigue and the postsurgical patient. In C. Norris (Ed.), *Concept clarification in nursing* (pp. 277–300). Rockville, MD: Aspen Systems.

Schmidt, S.P., & Shell, J.A. (1994). Lung cancer. In S.E. Otto (Ed.), *Oncology nursing* (pp. 303–339). St. Louis: Mosby.

Sigmund, D. (1994). Lung cancer. In J.H. Stein (Ed.), *Internal medicine* (4th ed.) (pp. 947–958). St. Louis: Mosby.

Chapter Six

Breast Cancer in Elderly Women

Beverly S. Reigle, PhD, RN

Introduction

Incidence and Mortality

The breast is the most prevalent site of cancer in women and second only to the lungs as the leading site of cancer deaths (American Cancer Society [ACS], 1999). ACS estimated that 175,000 women would develop breast cancer and that 43,300 would die of the disease in 1999. The five-year survival rate for local disease is 97%: 77% for regional and 22% for metastatic disease (ACS).

Risk Factors

The exact cause of breast cancer is not known. However, several factors have been identified as increasing one's risk for developing the disease, including gender, increased age, a family history of breast cancer, a personal history of the disease (Kelsey & Gammon, 1991), and biopsy-confirmed proliferative breast disease (Harris & Morrow, 1996). Of the factors found to increase one's risk, gender and age are the two most powerful determinants of breast cancer development (Fentiman, 1998). Ninety-nine percent of breast cancers are found in women (Moore, 1996), with 50% of the cases occurring in women over 65 years of age (Fentiman).

Age-Related Changes

Knowledge of age-related changes in the breasts is important to the effective performance of breast examinations. The female breast is primarily composed of glandular, fibrous, and adipose tissues (Bates, Bickley, & Hoekelman, 1995). The glandular tissue consists of approximately 10–20 lobes with a duct system that leads from the lobes to exit sites on the nipple. During the postmenopausal years, glandular tissue atrophies and is replaced by adipose tissue, causing a decrease in breast size. The ducts that surround the nipple assume a "firm stringy" (Bates et al., 1995, p. 318) consistency and are more palpable. Additionally, the suspensory ligaments (i.e., fibrous tissue) relax, allowing the breasts to hang loosely on the chest wall, and the inframammary ridge, located at the lower edge of the breasts, thickens. Following the process of menopausal involution, Gray (1985) described the breast as "a shriveled pendulous fold of skin" (p. 1583). Although such a description is not complimentary to the elderly female, the changes do have a positive impact in that the breasts are less dense, thus facilitating the detection of an abnormality.

The Gender Factor

Gender strongly implicates the woman's endocrine milieu. Hormonal influences that have been found to increase a woman's risk for breast cancer include early menarche (i.e., < 12 years old), late menopause (i.e., > 55 years old), nulliparity, and first pregnancy at age 30 or older (Fentiman, 1998). Based on a review of the literature, Fentiman noted that factors such as weight gain, endogenous estrogen, and hormone replacement therapy (HRT) increase a woman's risk of developing the disease depending on her menstrual status. For example, postmenopausal women with high levels of endogenous hormones are at increased risk of developing breast cancer. Additionally, postmenopausal women who are overweight face an increased risk of developing the disease. A woman's risk increases slightly if she has received HRT for more than five years. However, the risk of dying from the disease does not increase.

Genetic Factors

Genetic factors also have been found to play a significant role in the development of breast cancer. However, genetic mutations (e.g., BRCA1, BRCA2) only account for approximately 5%–10% of breast cancer cases (Fentiman, 1998). The lifetime risk of women who are gene carriers is 50%– 85% (National Cancer Institute [NCI], 1999b).

Dietary Factors

Researchers have theorized that diet influences a woman's risk for breast cancer. Of the factors investigated, a moderate level of alcohol consumption is the most well-established risk factor (Hunter & Willett, 1996). The complexity of dealing with this finding revolves around the protective cardiovascular effects that one or two alcoholic drinks afford. Thus, promoting total abstinence may not be the most effective approach (Fentiman, 1998). Researchers also have identified increased dietary fat intake as a potential risk factor for the disease. However, based on a literature review, Hunter and Willett noted that dietary fat as a risk factor has not been supported by prospective studies, even with 10 years of follow-up.

Based on our current knowledge of breast cancer development and, in particular, the discovery of breast cancer susceptibility genes, the hope of preventing and effectively eliminating breast cancer exists. However, at this time, early detection remains the primary method of combating the disease (ACS, 1999).

Screening

Assessment

The nurse is instrumental in promoting breast health behaviors. However, interventions that aid in performing these behaviors must be based on appropriate assessment data and must be collaboratively planned and implemented with the elderly patient. Specific subjective data that should be addressed include

- A history of comorbid conditions
- Use of HRT and length of time used
- Family history of breast cancer
- Personal history of breast cancer or breast problems
- Last mammogram and frequency pattern
- Last clinical breast examination (CBE) and frequency pattern
- Breast self-examination (BSE) frequency and proficiency
- Perceived susceptibility to and severity of breast cancer
- Perceived value of mammography, CBE, and BSE
- Perceived ability to utilize mammography and CBE and to perform BSE
- Perceived barriers to utilizing the three early-detection methods (e.g., forgetfulness, transportation, cost, lack of knowledge of screening guidelines, lack of knowledge of how to perform BSE)
- Cognitive abilities, particularly reading ability
- Sociocultural background.

Some healthcare providers suggest that data regarding age at menarche, number of pregnancies, number of live births, and age at first birth should be obtained from all women, regardless of age (Morrow, 1996).

Physical examination data that is pertinent to the promotion of breast health behaviors include

- Visual acuity
- Sensory perception, particularly in the fingerpads
- Musculoskeletal integrity
- Cognitive abilities, particularly comprehension and memory
- Comorbid conditions that may influence the practice of breast health behaviors (e.g., severe cardiovascular or respiratory disease that produces impaired activity tolerance).

Nursing Diagnoses and Plan of Care

Nursing diagnoses are based on a patient's specific assessment data (i.e., not standardized), are collaboratively developed with the patient, and have a healthcare response and etiology that can be modified or changed by the independent actions of the nurse. Two nursing care plans follow, and additional nursing diagnoses are suggested.

Nursing diagnosis: Health management deficit (mammography and/or CBE) related to lack of knowledge about breast cancer screening methods.

Supporting data: Elderly female who reports not having routine CBE or mammogram, expresses a lack of knowledge about mammograms and/or CBE (e.g., recommended frequency, what a mammogram or CBE entails, purpose of screening methods)

Goal: The patient will obtain a CBE and/or mammogram. If the nurse anticipates seeing the patient on a routine basis, the goal should be that the patient will obtain annual CBE and/or mammogram.

Predicted outcomes: The patient will (a) verbalize recommended CBE and/or mammogram frequency, (b) verbalize importance of early-detection methods and value of mammography and/or CBE methods for detecting breast cancer early, and (c) verbalize established date for contacting mammography facility and or primary healthcare provider.

Interventions:
- Instruct about personal risk factors for breast cancer.

- Discuss the importance of early detection and the value of mammogram and/or CBE as early-detection methods.
- Discuss recommended frequency of mammogram and CBE.
- Provide list of local mammography facilities that are American College of Radiology certified and telephone numbers (specify those facilities nearest patient's residence).
- Provide list of local primary care providers and telephone numbers.
- Establish an agreed-upon date for contacting the mammography facility and/or primary healthcare provider.
- Provide brochures (e.g., ACS or NCI literature appropriate for age, reading ability, and ethnicity) on mammography and CBE.
- Refer to local ACS for additional information (provide telephone number).

Evaluation: Formatively, note the patient's response to each intervention and determine effectiveness. Summatively, determine whether all predicted outcomes were met at the end of the session. At the next visit, if appropriate, determine if the goal was achieved. If future visits are not anticipated (e.g., acute-care facilities), establish a method of follow-up.

Nursing diagnosis: Health management deficit (BSE) related to lack of knowledge of the BSE behavior.

Supporting data: Elderly female who reports she has had annual mammogram and CBE reports that she does not do BSE and does not know how to perform the examination.

Goal: The patient will perform monthly BSE.

Predicted outcomes: The patient will (a) state purpose and benefits of BSE, (b) state frequency and timing of BSE, (c) state changes to note during BSE and importance of reporting changes to healthcare provider, (d) demonstrate the BSE technique correctly, (e) demonstrate ability to identify changes in breast consistency using a breast model, and (f) verbalize intent to perform monthly BSE.

Interventions:

- Discuss risk factors of breast cancer, the importance of early detection, and the benefits of BSE.
- Discuss frequency and timing of BSE, changes to note during examination, and importance of reporting changes to healthcare provider.
- Demonstrate the BSE technique (inspection and palpation), and during the demonstration emphasize
  - The purpose of the four positions when observing for changes in the breasts
  - The purpose of a correct supine position
  - Use of fingerpads
  - Parameters for breast coverage
  - Importance of using a systematic method
  - Use of three levels of pressure
  - Importance of maintaining fingerpads on breast when moving from one area to another
  - Importance of viewing each breast as a mirror-image of the other and comparing appearance and tissue consistency.
- Suggest modifications in positions (if range of motion [ROM] of upper extremities decreased or if unable to assume a supine position).
- Assist patient to identify changes in breast consistency using breast models, and allow sufficient time for practice.
- Suggest the use of a magnifying or illuminated mirror for patients with decreased visual acuity (Maddox, 1991).

- Provide BSE calendar for monthly BSE recording.
- Provide BSE brochure for future reference (if appropriate, use brochure with large print) (see Figure 6.1).

Evaluation: Formatively, note the patient's response to each intervention and determine effectiveness. Summatively, determine whether all predicted outcomes were met at the end of the session. At the next visit, if appropriate, determine if the goal was met. If future visits are not anticipated (e.g., acute-care facilities), establish a method of follow-up.

Other diagnoses may include the same response (i.e., health management deficit) with different etiologies. Examples of other etiologies are lack of perceived susceptibility for breast cancer, fear of being diagnosed with breast cancer, lack of motivation for performing BSE, decreased physical ability (specify), decreased BSE self-efficacy, difficulty remembering to perform BSE, and difficulty remembering to schedule routine CBE and mammogram.

Diagnosis of Breast Cancer in Elderly Women

Background

Breast cancer is diagnosed in more than 90% of elderly women based on the discovery of a palpable lump (Law et al., 1996). The most common type of breast cancer in all women is infiltrating or invasive ductal carcinoma, accounting for 70%–80% of all tumors (NCI, 1999a). In women older than 68, it accounts for 77%–85% of all tumors (Law et al.).

The incidence of papillary and mucinous carcinomas increases as a woman's age increases. However, the incidence of lobular carcinoma in situ, comedo, medullary, and inflammatory carcinomas decreases. Interestingly, the incidence of ductal carcinoma in situ (DCIS) increases until age 75, after which it decreases.

Tumors in women older than 70 years of age are more commonly estrogen receptor (ER) positive than those found in younger women, and according to data obtained from 50 state tumor registries, tumors in the elderly were more likely to be progesterone receptor (PR) positive than those in younger women. The ER and PR results are helpful factors in determining treatment options. Additionally, tumors in postmenopausal women tend to have a lower proliferative index than in premenopausal women (Bellet, Alonso, & Ojeda, 1995).

According to Fleming and Fleming (1994), breast cancer is usually diagnosed at a more advanced clinical stage in older women than younger women. Based on a review of several retrospective studies and data sources, Bellet et al. (1995) found that among patients with breast cancer who were older than 75 years of age, stages III, IV, and unknown stages were registered more frequently than for younger patients. Wanebo et al. (1997) found that early detection of preinvasive cancers occurred significantly less often in elderly patients than in younger patients. Although these studies provide some insight regarding tumor characteristics in older patients, documentation regarding stage and grade of breast tumors is often not available (Bellet et al.; Busch et al., 1996). Thus, determining the efficacy of treatment options in the elderly is a major health issue.

Assessment

History: As noted earlier, a palpable mass is often the presenting problem for older women diagnosed with breast cancer. If a woman reports finding a breast abnormality, a careful analysis of the finding should be made. For example, determine the location of the

Figure 6.1. How to Do a Breast Self-Exam

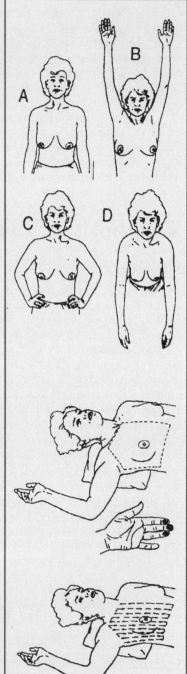

Observing your breasts in front of the mirror:

1. Remove all clothing from your waist up and stand in front of a mirror large enough to view both of your breasts at the same time.
2. Use four different positions while standing in front of the mirror to help you recognize changes in your breasts.
   A. Stand with arms relaxed at your sides.
   B. Place arms overhead and turn to view each side.
   C. Place hands on hips, press hands in, and turn.
   D. Bend forward with arms out straight or supported on table.
3. Look for any change in size, shape, color, and symmetry and texture of your breast, such as
   - Dimpling
   - Scaliness, especially around the nipple
   - Increase in size
   - Puckering or change in the shape and contour of the breast
   - Change in the direction that the nipple(s) point or a pulling to one side
   - Redness
   - Inversion of the nipple (pulling in)
4. Gently squeeze your nipple once, and note any discharge or fluid that may occur.
   - Observe for discharge unrelated to breast-feeing.
   - Observe for discharge that occurs spontaneously or that occurs without squeezing the nipple.

Examining your breasts in the lying position:

The most effective way to feel for changes in the breasts is in the lying position. This position helps spread the breast across the chest wall.

1. To feel the left side:
   - Place a small towel or pad behind the left shoulder blade.
   - Place the left arm behind your head.
   - Know the borders of the breast so that you thoroughly check all of your breast. Upper border is the collar bone, middle border is the breast bone, side border is an imaginary line from under the arm to the bra line, and the bottom border is the bra line.
   - Use the fingerpads (not fingertips) of the three middle fingers of your right hand to feel the breasts. To help the fingerpads move over the breasts, you may want to use lotion or powder.

(Continued on next page)

Figure 6.1. How to Do a Breast Self-Exam *(Continued)*

- Use a systematic method. A systematic method helps you know where to begin and end your examination, which is important for thorough coverage. The recommended methods are concentric circles or up-and-down lines (vertical strips).
- Use three levels of pressure beginning with light followed by medium and deep. Place your fingerpads at the beginning point (e.g., the 12 o'clock position when using the concentric circle method). Make three dime-size circular movements, staying at the same point and using all three levels of pressure. The deep pressure assists you to press against the chest wall.
- Release the pressure while keeping your fingerpads on the breast and move to the next area. Repeat the last two steps until the whole breast is checked, including the nipple area.

2. **To feel the right side:**
   - Use the same technique on the right side as described for the left side.
   - Compare what you feel in the right breast to what you felt in the left. For example, a firm ridge that provides support for the breast is a normal structure felt at the lower curve of each breast.

3. **Learn what your breasts feel like and what is normal for you. Feel for any changes, such as a thickened area, a lump, or a cluster of lumps or granule-like lumps.**
   - Report any changes to your healthcare professional right away. Know that your concerns are always valid and that any change that you observe or feel in your breast is worth reporting to your healthcare professional.
   - Remember the areas of your breast that have been diagnosed as fibrocystic or as having a benign condition (it helps to draw a picture of the breast and mark where the areas are). Become familiar with the way these areas feel so that you will be able to detect a change on future exams.

Examining your breasts in the shower:

   This position is optional but can be used in addition to the observation and lying down positions. Soap and/or water replaces the lotion or powder for each movement of the fingerpads on the breast. The method of feeling the breast is the same as the method described in the lying position. The changes to note and report are also the same as described in the lying position.

Note. From *Ohio Breast Cancer Screening Guide* (pp. 11–14), by the American Cancer Society–Ohio Division. Columbus, OH: Author. Copyright 1995 by the American Cancer Society–Ohio Division. Reprinted with permission.

abnormality, how long ago the abnormality was found, in what manner it was found, any change in the abnormality over time, and other symptoms associated with the abnormality. A clinical examination of the breast should be conducted, including a careful history and thorough physical examination of the breast. Essential information to obtain includes family history of breast cancer, personal history of breast cancer, history of breast biopsies (histology, if known), and hormonal factors that increase a woman's risk for breast cancer (e.g., use of HRT and duration of use).

Physical assessment: The physical examination should consist of a thorough inspection and palpation of the breasts. Adequate lighting, appropriate room temperature (i.e., not cold), and privacy should be ensured. With the patient disrobed from the waist up and arms relaxed at her side, inspect the breasts for symmetry in size (i.e., slight differences are expected, but note if difference is of recent onset) and shape (e.g., dimpling, bulges, retractions), and note color and texture of the skin (e.g., erythema, edema). Note that in older women the breasts often appear flaccid and droop due to the weakened ligaments and decreased subcutaneous tissue (Ludwick, 1988). Inspect the nipples for symmetry, retraction, ulceration, and eczematous changes (Morrow, 1996). Have the patient raise her arms to allow for better inspection of the lower half of the breasts and to press her hands on her hips to highlight subtle areas of retraction (Morrow). To further emphasize subtle changes, have her lean forward so that the breasts hang loosely. While in the sitting position with the flexed arm supported on the side examined, palpate the axillary and supraclavicular nodes. Axillary nodes that are small, soft, and mobile are not highly suspicious, and many women have them because of problems such as hangnails and minor arm abrasions. However, supraclavicular nodularity is not common and requires further evaluation. Additionally, while in the sitting position, palpate the breasts. Support the breast with one hand and, using the fingerpads of the index and two middle fingers, palpate the breasts. This position, in particular, aids in detecting lesions in the tail of the breast (Morrow).

Next, have the patient assume the supine position, place a small towel under the scapula on the side being examined, and raise the arm on the side being examined. Using a systematic approach (e.g., concentric circles or vertical method), palpate the area from the clavicle to the lower rib cage and from the sternum to the midclavicular line. With the fingerpads, make dime-sized circular movements using three levels of pressure (i.e., light, medium, and deep) at each site. Maintain the fingerpads on the breasts while moving from one site to another. If a mass is palpated, note if its density differs from surrounding tissue, if it is three dimensional, and if it occurs in the absence of other abnormalities of similar description. Note the location, size, character, and mobility of the mass. In addition, comparing the same areas in each breast assists in determining the need for further evaluation of a finding.

Finally, the nipple is gently compressed to detect discharge. If the patient has reported a history of discharge, the quadrants of the breast should be sequentially compressed and the nipple-areolar complex milked to ascertain the location of the discharge and whether it is confined to one duct (Winchester, 1996). Nipple discharge that is considered pathologic has the following clinical features (Winchester).

- Spontaneous
- Unilateral
- Confined to one duct
- Associated with a mass
- Bloody, serous, serosanguineous, or watery.

Generally, bloody discharge and a palpable mass are associated with invasive ductal carcinoma, whereas occult bleeding is more often associated with DCIS or papillary carcinoma. All of these are cancers are commonly found in older women.

All findings should be carefully documented. If an abnormality is found, the information should be reported to the appropriate healthcare provider. Unfortunately, palpable lesions in older women are more likely to be malignant (Muss, 1996).

Nursing/Collaborative Management

Diagnosis: A mammogram of both breasts often is recommended as the initial procedure following the detection of a palpable mass (Fentiman, 1998). In the event the mammography results are negative, Eberlein (1993) strongly urges further pathologic physical evaluation in older women. For a definitive diagnosis, a biopsy is required. The four techniques used for a palpable mass are fine-needle aspiration biopsy, core-cutting needle biopsy, excisional biopsy, and incisional biopsy (Foster, 1996). Often a two-step process is employed; that is, a time interval exists between the biopsy and the treatment. This time interval allows the healthcare provider and patient to have a discussion about treatment options (Foster). However, depending on the stage of the disease, treatment options may be limited. Even so, the time span allows the patient to participate in the decision-making process and, if desired, to receive a second opinion.

ER and PR assays need to be performed on the biopsy specimen to help determine prognosis and to provide information on the likely response to endocrine therapy. The absence of these tumor receptors is predictive of early recurrence and poor survival, and their presence predicts the likelihood of a beneficial response to endocrine therapy (Fuqua, 1996). Fuqua noted that ER- and PR-positive tumors are likely to be more differentiated and diploid and have a lower proliferative rate. This information is very important for older women, because they tend to derive more benefit from tamoxifen, an endocrine therapy, than women less than 50 years old (Osborne, Clark, & Ravdin, 1996).

Nursing Diagnoses and Plan of Care

Although the physician is expected to provide a full explanation of the biopsy procedure, the nurse should determine the patient's understanding of the information as well as reinforce the information. The following are potential diagnoses based on assessment of the patient's emotional status, her understanding of the biopsy procedure and post-biopsy care, and her response to making a decision about treatment.

Nursing diagnosis: Anxiety related to lack of knowledge about biopsy procedure or anxiety related to inadequate understanding about biopsy procedure.

Supporting data: The patient has breast biopsy scheduled and expresses anxiety about breast biopsy, has no previous breast biopsy experience, states she is not familiar with biopsy procedure or verbalizes inaccurate information about procedure, reports inability to relax, and exhibits restless movements.

Goal: The patient will express peace of mind about procedure for breast biopsy.

Predicted outcomes: The patient will verbalize components of breast biopsy procedure.

Interventions:
- Explain procedure using appropriate visuals such as a video of the procedure (Northouse, Tocco, & West, 1997).
- Provide adequate time for questions.
- Provide large-print breast-biopsy pamphlet.
- Provide calm support without false reassurance (Northouse et al.).

Evaluation: Formatively, determine response to explanation of procedure and effectiveness of handouts. Summatively, determine if predicted outcomes and goal have been met.

Nursing diagnosis: Decisional conflict about treatment choices related to complexity and impact of breast cancer treatment options.

Supporting data: The patient receives breast cancer diagnosis, has been informed by physician of treatment options, expresses concern about impact of decision on life, expresses difficulty choosing treatment, and expresses difficulty understanding options.

Goal: The patient will express satisfaction with decision about breast cancer treatment.

Predicted outcomes: The patient will (a) verbalize advantages and disadvantages of treatment options and (b) involve family or identified support person in decision-making process.

Interventions:

- Encourage verbalization of treatment options.
- Clarify misconceptions and/or refer to physician if appropriate.
- Encourage verbalization of advantages and disadvantages of options.
- Encourage discussion of treatment options with family, significant other, or identified support person.
- Recommend and, if agreed upon, contact ACS for a Reach to Recovery or Reconstruction Education for National Understanding (RENU) volunteer to visit.

Evaluation: Formatively, determine effectiveness of each intervention. Summatively, determine if predicted outcomes and goals were met.

Current Treatment of Breast Cancer in Elderly Women

Background

Treatment of elderly patients with breast cancer depends on multiple factors such as functional ability, concomitant diseases, socioeconomic resources, transportation access, and compliance (Busch et al., 1996). Comorbid conditions adversely affect survival and must be considered in determining treatment. However, Newschaffer, Penberthy, Desch, Retchin, and Wittemore (1996) found that comorbidity did not explain the age-related patterns in the initial treatment of elderly patients with breast cancer. In support of this finding, Law et al. (1996), following a review of several studies, found that age independently influenced treatment decisions in elderly women regardless of the severity of concurrent illnesses. For example, they found that less definitive surgery did not always correlate with the severity of concurrent medical conditions. However, they also noted that between 13% and 55% of patients died of causes other than breast cancer.

In reviewing cancer registry records for women 66 years of age and older who were diagnosed with nonmetastatic, invasive breast cancer, Newschaffer et al. (1996) found that patients who were older than 74 years of age were, initially, less likely to be treated surgically than women ages 66–74 years. Women ages 85 years and older who were surgically treated were less likely to receive a modified radical mastectomy than women younger than 85 (i.e., one-third less likely). Additionally, women who were older than 74 years of age and who received breast-conserving surgery (e.g., lumpectomy) were less likely to receive adjuvant radiation therapy than women ages 66–74. However, in a review of the literature, Law et al. (1996) found that women ages 65 years and older tolerated radiation as well as those younger than age 65 and had similar 10-year survival rates. Regarding surgery, Muss (1996) reported that no evidence exists that suggests that older women with breast cancer have a higher rate of surgical complications than younger women. Thus, elderly women who are able to tolerate standard therapy for breast cancer are not always provided the option but should be.

Another primary therapy, considered by some to be appropriate for elderly women, is tamoxifen. The efficacy of tamoxifen, as a primary treatment, has been investigated, and according to Fentiman (1998), tamoxifen alone is inadequate treatment for breast cancer, particularly for elderly women who do not have severe comorbidity. Overall, care of the elderly patient with breast cancer should include a "plan for long-term control of the cancer (cure), maintenance of a maximum level of patient independence, freedom of symptoms, and maintenance of personal dignity and life-style" (Wanebo et al., 1997, p. 581). This implies that, unless contraindicated, elderly women should have the choice of similar treatment options that younger women have.

Standard Treatment for Stage I and II Breast Cancer

Stage I and II invasive breast cancers are most often treated with either a modified radical mastectomy (i.e., total mastectomy with axillary dissection) or lumpectomy and axillary node dissection followed by radiation therapy (Law et al., 1996). Often, women older than 70 are viewed as accepting mastectomy more quickly than younger women and not tolerating radiotherapy well. However, Sandison, Gold, Wright, and Jones (1996) found that of 38 women who were ages 70 years and older and chose their own treatment, 31 selected breast conservation (i.e., complete local excision, radiotherapy, and tamoxifen), and only 4 chose mastectomy. Of the four that chose mastectomy, three stated that their doctors had highly recommended it, and one stated that radiotherapy would be too much trouble. At 12 months, only 2 of the 38 women were disappointed in their choice (e.g., concerned about the initial skin erythema following radiotherapy).

Treatment for Early-Stage Breast Cancer in Elderly Women

Modified radical mastectomy: Patients who have modified radical mastectomies undergo general anesthesia and are hospitalized for approximately one to two days. Drains are placed beneath the skin flap and remain for approximately three to five days postsurgery (Goodman & Harte, 1990) or, if discharged home, are removed at the one-week follow-up visit (Naumann, 1999). A pressure dressing typically is applied. If reconstruction is not performed at the time of the mastectomy, some surgeons apply a dressing that contains a sterile prosthesis supported by a surgical brassiere. Protective measures of the arm on the mastectomy side begin immediately after surgery to prevent lymphedema and infection. Incremental arm exercises (e.g., initially, squeezing a rubber ball) begin one day postoperatively (Barr, 1990). With early discharge, the patient or caregiver is taught wound care, drain care, pain management, arm precautions, and arm exercises.

Reconstructive surgery is an important option for women who are eligible for the procedure. The surgeon should discuss the option of reconstruction prior to the mastectomy (Ellis, 1994). If eligible, she should be informed of the reconstructive choices. Reconstruction can be accomplished by a prosthetic implant, tissue expansion, or flap procedures, and it can be done at the time of the mastectomy or much later (Ellis). Importantly, the woman should be well informed of the advantages and disadvantages of each. If comorbid conditions exist, assess appropriately.

In addition to the modified radical mastectomy, elderly patients are often given tamoxifen for at least two to five years if they have an invasive breast tumor that is larger than 1 centimeter in diameter (Law et al., 1996). Tamoxifen is well tolerated by older women. In general, studies indicate that postmenopausal women with early-stage breast cancer respond well to adjuvant hormonal therapy (e.g., tamoxifen), whereas premenopausal women with early-stage breast cancer have a better response to adjuvant chemotherapy (Law et al.). However, chemotherapy may be an option for elderly women who are at high risk for recurrence (i.e., are node-positive and have tumors that are larger than 2 centimeters and hormone receptor-negative).

Breast conservation: A lumpectomy, which involves a local excision, is the most common breast-conserving surgery performed (Harris & Morrow, 1996). At the time of the local excision, axillary nodes are dissected to achieve regional control and to assist in determining prognosis and the role and type of adjuvant therapy (Recht, 1993). Breast-conserving surgery often is performed in a same-day surgical setting. Drains usually are inserted, particularly with axillary dissection. Care is similar to that provided to patients who have had a modified radical mastectomy: arm exercises, lymphedema prevention, wound care, pain management, and arm infection precautions.

Radiation therapy is initiated approximately three to four weeks postoperatively (Carlson, 1991). The whole breast is tangentially irradiated at a dose of 45–50 Gy delivered over 4.5–5 weeks (Harris & Morrow, 1996). Axillary node irradiation is typically performed if the patient has greater than three positive nodes at level I/II. Supraclavicular irradiation also may be performed, but this treatment is debatable. The most common side effects of radiation therapy are skin reactions; dealing with pains in the breast, chest wall, or axilla; breast edema; and fatigue.

Assessment

Preoperatively, assess the patient's and significant other's emotional status and knowledge of the procedure and postoperative care. Following surgery, perform typical postoperative assessment (e.g., assess vital signs according to protocol, intake/output). Related to breast surgery, specifically assess
• Wound and drainage catheters
• Arm on side of mastectomy
• Level of pain
• Emotional response to surgery (e.g., body image).

Collaborative Care

Collaborative care consists of the following.
• Elevate and slightly flex the arm on side of mastectomy.
• Position on unaffected side.
• Implement arm precautions, and display precautions for other healthcare professionals.
• Provide pain medication on a regular basis, and perform wound care (i.e., according to protocol).
• Empty drainage container and report if > 200 cc in eight hours (Carlson, 1991)
• Administer medications as ordered, and inform of follow-up visits (e.g., usually one week postsurgery and on routine basis for lifetime).

Nursing Diagnoses and Plan of Care

Several nursing diagnoses are relevant to surgeries, in general. However, some of those specific to breast cancer surgery with early discharge are discussed.

Nursing diagnosis: Risk for infection related to lack of knowledge of postsurgical wound care.

Supporting data: The patient undergoing breast cancer surgery expresses no knowledge of postsurgical wound care and has concomitant conditions that increase risk for infection (e.g., diagnosed with diabetes and rheumatoid arthritis and taking corticosteroids or methotrexate).

Goal: The patient will not exhibit signs and symptoms of infection.

Predicted outcomes: The patient will (a) verbalize procedure for wound care, (b) verbalize signs and symptoms of infection, (c) demonstrate care of drains and dressing, and (d) demonstrate care of surgical site.

Interventions: Based on a modification of McCorkle, Baird, and Grant's protocol as cited in Naumann (1999)
• Instruct on dressing change according to protocol (e.g., change dressing when soiled and replace with dry gauze)

- Instruct on care of drain sites and drainage container (if in place).
- Instruct to take sponge baths until drains and sutures/staples are removed, and keep sites dry.
- Instruct on follow-up visit (e.g., 7–10 days postoperatively) when drains and sutures/staples are removed.
- Instruct on signs and symptoms of infection or excessive bleeding.
- Allow time for questions and answers.
- Supervise hands-on practice with care of drainage container and dressing.

Evaluation: Formatively, determine effectiveness of each instruction and or intervention. Summatively, determine if predicted outcomes and goal were met.

Nursing diagnosis: Health management deficit (arm exercises/care) related to lack of knowledge of lymphedema prevention and methods to increase arm mobility.

Supporting data: The patient had breast cancer surgery with axillary dissection and states no knowledge of how to prevent lymphedema.

Goal: The patient will have minimal or no lymphedema.

Predicted outcomes: The patient will (a) verbalize exercises/care to prevent lymphedema and increase mobility, (b) demonstrate exercises to prevent lymphedema and increase mobility, and (c) verbalize rationale for exercises.

Interventions: Primarily based on Barr (1990)

- Instruct on arm positioning (i.e., elevate arm several times/day) and pumping exercises (postoperative day 1–4 or while drains are in place).
- Instruct on pendulum exercises, shoulder shrugs, and shoulder retraction (postoperative day 4–9).
- Instruct on wall ladder, wand, and ROM exercises (postoperative day 10–6 weeks and after sutures are removed).
- Instruct on resistive exercises after six weeks postoperatively.
- Instruct on not overtiring the arm and, if aching occurs, to lie down and elevate the arm (Thiadens, 1994).
- Instruct to avoid saunas and strenuous exertion (Petrek & Lerner, 1996).
- Encourage use of antilymphedema compression garment or bandage when performing vigorous aerobic exercises (Petrek & Lerner).
- Inform about ENCORE Program (a YWCA program that provides floor and pool exercises).

Evaluation: Formatively, determine effectiveness of each intervention (e.g., response to instruction about positioning of arm). Summatively, determine if predicted outcomes and goal were met. Again, goal will most likely be noted by healthcare provider or homecare nurse.

Nursing diagnosis: Risk for infection related to lack of knowledge of arm precautions after mastectomy or axillary dissection.

Supporting data: The patient had breast cancer surgery with axillary dissection and expresses no knowledge of susceptibility to infection related to affected arm and no knowledge of ways to prevent infection in affected arm.

Goal: The patient will exhibit no signs or symptoms of infection.

Predicted outcomes: The patient will (a) verbalize arm precautions and (b) verbalize signs and symptoms of infection and importance of reporting to physician.

Interventions: Primarily based on Petrek and Lerner (1996)

- Instruct about signs and symptoms of infection and to report abnormalities to physician.
- Instruct to avoid vaccinations, venipuncture, IV administrations, and blood pressure monitoring in affected arm.
- Instruct to avoid puncturing or injuring skin on affected hand and arm (e.g., maintain meticulous nail and cuticle care).

- Instruct to avoid wearing constricting sleeves or jewelry and to wear a padded bra strap.
- Instruct to avoid heat, sunburns, and tanning beds.
- Instruct to avoid smoking with affected arm (Barr, 1990).
- Instruct to wear protective gloves when washing dishes or gardening (Barr).
- Instruct to prevent excoriation of skin by using lotion liberally and avoiding harsh detergents (Barr).
- Encourage to contact ACS for Reach to Recovery literature and to talk with volunteer.
- Encourage to have medical alert information on person.

Evaluation: Formatively, determine the effectiveness of each instruction. Summatively, determine if predicted outcomes were met. Healthcare provider should evaluate goal over time.

Nursing diagnosis: Body image disturbance related to perceived loss of femininity after mastectomy.

Supporting data: The patient has had removal of a breast and expresses fear of rejection by others and feelings of loss of femininity. The patient may not view or discuss mastectomy and may have hair loss from chemotherapy.

Goal: The patient will express positive perceptions of body and self.

Predicted outcomes: The patient will (a) look at and touch mastectomy site, (b) verbalize reframing of perceptions of self, and (c) involve significant other in acceptance process.

Interventions:
- Encourage verbalization of perceptions regarding loss of breast.
- Discuss prosthetic options, if reconstruction is not an option or not desired, and provide information on approved breast prosthesis.
- Discuss reconstruction options and refer to appropriate provider if desired.
- Encourage open communication with significant other and involve in acceptance process.
- Suggest participation in Look Good . . . Feel Better program (ACS program that provides wigs, make-up tips, etc. for patients with cancer).
- Encourage looking at and touching mastectomy site (Johnson & Klein, 1994).
- Encourage reframing of perceptions (e.g., body is healthier and more vibrant).
- Provide list of support groups (e.g., Reach to Recovery).

Evaluation: Formatively, determine effectiveness of each intervention. Summatively, determine if predicted outcomes and goal were met.

Nursing diagnosis: Health management deficit (BSE/mastectomy) related to lack of knowledge about detecting changes in mastectomy site and contralateral breast.

Supporting data: The patient had breast cancer surgery and expresses a lack of knowledge about detecting changes in mastectomy site and a lack of knowledge about assessing unaffected breast.

Goal: The patient will perform monthly BSE of contralateral breast and routine assessment of mastectomy site.

Predicted outcomes: The same objectives for performing BSE as stated earlier are appropriate. In addition, the following are appropriate objectives postmastectomy: (a) verbalize purpose and method for examining chest on mastectomy side, (b) demonstrate mastectomy assessment technique, and (c) verbalize changes to report to physician.

Interventions: The same interventions for teaching BSE are appropriate, with the addition of the following.
- Instruct to examine the entire chest wall on affected side from clavicle to lower rib and axilla to sternum and note scar.
- Instruct to note and report any changes such as rash, pimple-like area, color change, edema, or lump.
- Demonstrate palpation method called "stripping," in which tissue between each rib is palpated horizontally (ACS-Ohio Division, 1995).

Evaluation: Formatively, determine effectiveness of each intervention (e.g., instruction and demonstration). Summatively, determine if predicted outcomes and goals were met. The goal may be evaluated by healthcare provider or by routine follow-up calls.

Standard Therapy for Advanced Breast Cancer

Hormonal therapy is a standard therapy for advanced breast cancer. Tamoxifen is considered the first-line therapy in women with ER-positive tumors or tumors with unknown receptor status (Law et al., 1996). However, the response is greater in certain sites such as soft tissue masses and bone. As discussed earlier, tamoxifen is tolerated by the majority of women. However, an association with endometrial cancer has been found (Aikin, 1996). Thus, women should be encouraged to report any vaginal bleeding and obtain yearly pelvic exams.

Second-line hormone therapy such as Megace® (Bristol-Myers Squibb Oncology, Princeton, NJ) may be instituted, but the response rate and duration are usually lower than for tamoxifen. A new hormonal therapy for advanced breast cancer is Femara®(Novartis, East Hanover, NJ). It is used in postmenopausal women who have previously received tamoxifen or another antiestrogen therapy and whose cancers are no longer controlled with such therapy (Novartis, 1997).

Chemotherapy may be used as a first-line treatment, particularly with women who have visceral metastasis, or it may be used when hormonal therapy is no longer effective (Law et al., 1996). In selected patients, chemotherapy may be an option over hormonal therapy due to the shorter response time (Law et al.). The combination of cyclophosphamide, methotrexate, and 5-fluorouracil is commonly used (Muss, 1996). Although doxorubicin has a high response rate (Law et al.), its cardiotoxicity must be considered in elderly patients, especially those at risk for congestive heart failure (Muss). Interestingly, Ibrahim, Frye, Buzdar, Walters, and Hortobagyi (1996) found that doxorubicin given for metastatic breast disease was tolerated as well by women older than 65 years of age as women younger than 65 years. However, mitoxantrone is another chemotherapeutic option that has proven efficacy and is less toxic than doxorubicin (Law et al.). In addition to less cardiotoxicity, it causes less nausea and vomiting and less alopecia (Muss).

The care of patients undergoing chemotherapy and radiation therapy is beyond the scope of this chapter. Please refer to the chapter on symptom management (Chapter 10) for nursing interventions that address problems common to individuals experiencing cancer.

Conclusion

Elderly women have been found to respond as well to standard therapy for breast cancer as younger women. Their survival rates are similar. However, as presented in this chapter, elderly women have frequently been provided fewer treatment options than younger women and some are suboptimally treated. Additionally, screening and treatment guidelines for elderly women frequently have not been based on rigorous scientific investigation. Thus, studies are needed in all disciplines to adequately provide care for this growing population.

References

Aikin, J.L. (1996). Tamoxifen in perspective: Benefits, side effects, and toxicities. In K.H. Dow (Ed.), *Contemporary issues in breast cancer* (pp. 59–68). Boston: Jones and Bartlett.

American Cancer Society. (1999). *Cancer facts and figures—1999*. Atlanta: Author.

American Cancer Society-Ohio Division. (1995). *Triple touch program*. Columbus, OH: Author.

Barr, D. (1990). Postmastectomy exercises. *Innovations in Oncology Nursing, 5*(3), 5–8.

Bates, B., Bickley, L.S., & Hoekelman, R.A. (1995). *A guide to physical examination and history taking: A guide to clinical thinking* (6th ed.). Philadelphia: Lippincott-Raven.

Bellet, M., Alonso, C., & Ojeda, B. (1995). Breast cancer in the elderly. *Postgraduate Medical Journal, 71*, 658–664.

Busch, E., Kemeny, M., Fremgen, A., Osteen, R.T., Winchester, D.P., & Clive, R.E. (1996). Patterns of breast cancer care in the elderly. *Cancer, 78*, 101–111.

Carlson, J. (1991). Breast cancer. In S.E. Otto (Ed.), *Oncology nursing* (pp. 77–96). St. Louis: Mosby.

Eberlein, T.J. (1993). Breast cancer surgery. In D.F. Hayes (Ed.), *Atlas of breast cancer* (pp. 5.2–5.17). London: Wolfe.

Ellis, C. (1994). Breast reconstruction after mastectomy. *Innovations in Oncology Nursing, 10*, 2–8, 26.

Fentiman, I.S. (1998). *Detection and treatment of breast cancer*. London: Martin Dunitz.

Fleming, I.D., & Fleming, M.D. (1994). Breast cancer in elderly women. *Cancer, 74*, 2160–2164.

Foster, R.S. (1996). Biopsy techniques. In J.R. Harris, M.E. Lippman, M. Morrow, & S. Hellman (Eds.), *Diseases of the breast* (pp. 133–138). Philadelphia: Lippincott-Raven.

Fuqua, S.A.W. (1996). Estrogen and progesterone receptors and breast cancer. In J.R. Harris, M.E. Lippman, M. Morrow, & S. Hellman (Eds.), *Diseases of the breast* (pp. 261–271). Philadelphia: Lippincott-Raven.

Goodman, M., & Harte, N. (1990). Breast cancer. In S.L. Groenwald, M.H. Frogge, M. Goodman, & C.H. Yarbro (Eds.), *Cancer nursing: Principles and practice* (pp. 722–750) Boston: Jones and Bartlett.

Gray, H. (1985). *Anatomy of the human body* (30th ed.). Philadelphia: Lea & Febiger.

Harris, J.R., & Morrow, M. (1996). Local management of invasive breast cancer. In J.R. Harris, M.E. Lippman, M. Morrow, & S. Hellman (Eds.), *Diseases of the breast* (pp. 487–547). Philadelphia: Lippincott-Raven.

Hunter, D.J., & Willett, W.C. (1996). Dietary factors. In J.R. Harris, M.E. Lippman, M. Morrow, & S. Hellman (Eds.), *Diseases of the breast* (pp. 201–212). Philadelphia: Lippincott-Raven.

Ibrahim, N.K., Frye, D.K., Buzdar, A.U., Walters, R.S., & Hortobagyi, G.N. (1996). Doxorubicin-based chemotherapy in elderly patients with metastatic breast cancer. *Archives of Internal Medicine, 156*, 882–888.

Johnson, J., & Klein, L. (1994). Enhancing sexuality and self-esteem after a breast cancer diagnosis. *Innovation in Oncology Nursing, 10*, 39–42.

Kelsey, J.L., & Gammon, M.D. (1991). The epidemiology of breast cancer. *CA: A Cancer Journal for Clinicians, 41*, 146–165.

Law, T.M., Hesketh, P.J., Porter, K.A., Lawn-Tsao, L., McAnaw, R., & Lopez, M.J. (1996). Breast cancer in elderly women. *Surgical Clinics of North America, 76*, 289–308.

Ludwick, R. (1988). Breast examination in the older adult. *Cancer Nursing, 11*, 99–102.

Maddox, M.A. (1991). The practice of breast self-examination among older women. *Oncology Nursing Forum, 18*, 1367–1371.

Moore, M. (1996). Special therapeutic problems. In J.R. Harris, M.E. Lippman, M. Morrow, & S. Hellman (Eds.), *Diseases of the breast* (pp. 859–863). Philadelphia: Lippincott-Raven.

Morrow, M. (1996). Physical examination of the breast. In J.R. Harris, M.E. Lippman, M. Morrow & S. Hellman (Eds.), *Diseases of the breast* (pp. 67–70). Philadelphia: Lippincott-Raven.

Muss, H.B. (1996). Breast cancer in older women. *Seminars in Oncology, 23*, 82–88.

National Cancer Institute. (1999a). Breast cancer. *PDQ for health professionals* [Online]. Available: http://cancernet.nci.nih.gov/clinpdq/soa/Breast_Cancer_Physician.html#2 [1999, November 9].

National Cancer Institute. (1999b). Genetic testing for breast cancer risk: It's your choice. *PDQ for health professionals* [Online]. Available: http://cancernet.nci.nih.gov/clinpdq/risk/Genetic_Testing_for_Breast_Cancer_Risk:_It's_your_choice.html [1999, November 9].

Naumann, P. (1999). Interventions for clients with breast disorders. In D.D. Ignatavicius, M.L. Workman, & M.A. Mishler (Eds.), *Medical-surgical nursing across the health care continuum* (pp. 1955–1979). Philadelphia: Saunders.

Newschaffer, C.J., Penberthy, L., Desch, C.E., Retchin, S.M., & Wittemore, M. (1996). The effect of age and comorbidity in the treatment of elderly women with nonmetastatic breast cancer. *Archives of Internal Medicine, 156*, 85–90.

Northouse, L.L., Tocco, K.M., & West, P. (1997). Coping with a breast biopsy: How healthcare professionals can help women and their husbands. *Oncology Nursing Forum, 24*, 473–480.

Novartis. (1997). *Understanding hormonal therapy*. East Hanover, NJ: Author.

Osborne, C.K., Clark, G.M., & Ravdin, P.M. (1996). Adjuvant systemic therapy of primary breast cancer. In J.R. Harris, M.E. Lippman, M. Morrow, & S. Hellman (Eds.), *Diseases of the breast* (pp. 548–578). Philadelphia: Lippincott-Raven.

Petrek, J.A.K., & Lerner, R. (1996). Lymphedema. In J.R. Harris, M.E. Lippman, M. Morrow, & S. Hellman (Eds.), *Diseases of the breast* (pp. 896–903). Philadelphia: Lippincott-Raven.

Recht, A. (1993). Radiotherapy techniques. In D.F. Hays (Ed.), *Atlas of breast cancer* (pp. 9.2–9.17). London: Wolfe.

Sandison, A.J.P., Gold, D.M., Wright, P., & Jones, P.A. (1996). Breast conservation or mastectomy: Treatment choice of women aged 70 years and older. *British Journal of Surgery, 83*, 994–996.

Thiadens, S.R.J. (1994). Prevention and treatment of lymphedema. *Innovations in Oncology Nursing, 10*, 63–64.

Wanebo, H.J., Cole, B., Chung, M., Vezeridis, M., Schepps, B., Fulton, J., & Bland, K. (1997). Is surgical management compromised in elderly patients with breast cancer? *Annals of Surgery, 224*, 579–589.

Winchester, D.P. (1996). Nipple discharge. In J.R. Harris, M.E. Lippman, M. Morrow, & S. Hellman (Eds.), *Diseases of the breast* (pp. 106–110). Philadelphia: Lippincott-Raven.

Chapter Seven

Treatment and Care of the Older Adult With Colorectal Cancer

Judith Schneider, MSN, RN, CRNH

Introduction

Colon and rectal cancers are the third most common cause of death from malignant disease in the United States. In 1998, an estimated 131,600 cases, accounting for approximately 11% of all new cancer diagnoses, were identified. Although the *colorectal* term will be used to discuss this disease, the individual numbers of colon versus rectal cancers are 95,600 and 36,000, respectively (American Cancer Society, 1998).

The diagnosis of colorectal cancers often is made late in the disease process, which leads to poor survival results. Usually a delay occurs between the onset of symptoms and diagnosis, even though a well-recognized premalignant lesion usually precedes this cancer. In many situations, patients delay in reporting symptoms such as rectal bleeding, change in bowel habits, and unexplained and persistent abdominal pain. In approximately 20% of patients undergoing surgery for colorectal cancers, the first presentation to the hospital was because of an emergency situation from a bowel obstruction. In most of these cases, reported symptoms occurred so late that the cancer already was well advanced (Hardcastle, 1997).

Parker, Tong, Bolden, and Wingo (1996) noted that the high incidence of colorectal cancers should justify the need for screening as part of routine care for all adults beginning at age 50. Screening should begin earlier for those people with first-degree relatives with colorectal cancer. The identification of high-risk groups, the demonstrated slow growth of primary lesions, the better survival of individuals with early-stage lesions, and the simplicity and accuracy of screening tests all point to the potential benefit of a thorough screening program.

Epidemiology

Within the United States, males and females have a similar rate of occurrence of colorectal cancer. The incidence significantly increases in people over age 50 and declines somewhat after age 75. African Americans and Caucasian Americans display similar patterns of occurrence, while the incidence in Native Americans is reported as less than half that of Caucasian Americans (American Cancer Society, 1998).

Etiology

The cause of colorectal cancer is unknown. However, research has revealed several factors that may impact the development of colorectal cancer.

Diet

Although under investigation, several elements in the daily diet of Americans are linked to gastrointestinal cancers. Excess fat seems to be the main culprit in promoting many diseases. Fat is being recognized as a promoter rather than a carcinogen in colorectal cancer. The mechanism of how fat influences the development of cancer still is uncertain, but several hypotheses link ingested food and length of time that it is in contact with the bowel mucosa as an initiating factor for the development of a malignancy. This gives credence to the theory that a diet high in fiber reduces the risk of malignancy formation by reducing the time the gut is exposed to carcinogenic food substances (Cohen, Minsky, & Schilsky, 1993).

Genetic Factors

Genetic factors play a significant role in identifying individuals who may be at increased risk. Approximately 10%–15% of people diagnosed with colorectal cancers have first-degree relatives who have had the disease. Familial adenomatosis polyposis is an inherited condition that greatly increases the risk of colorectal cancer. Other predisposing syndromes, such as ulcerative colitis and Crohn's disease, have been associated with the development of malignant disease of the bowel. Inflammatory bowel disorders over time may cause dysplasia, and as they progress, the probability of cancer increases.

Alcohol Consumption

Giovannucci et al. (1995) identified a two-fold increase in the risk of colon cancer when alcohol was consumed daily. Heavy drinkers of all types of alcoholic beverages are at increased risk of cancers of various types, including colorectal cancer (American Cancer Society, 1996).

Clinical Features

Obtaining a thorough history with an in-depth focus on the bowel when the chief complaint includes intestinal irregularity is important to identify clinical features of colon or rectal cancers. The most common sites of lesions of colorectal cancers, the percentage of occurrence, and the associated symptoms are
- Rectum (40%–50%): Changes in bowel habits, tenesmus, bright red blood, and severe pain in the groin, labia, scrotum, penis, and radiation down the legs
- Descending and sigmoid colon (20%–35%): Changes in bowel habits, bright red bleeding, constipation, rectal pressure, incomplete evacuation of stool, feelings of fullness, and gas pains
- Transverse colon (8%): Bloody stools, palpable masses, change in bowel habits, and possible obstruction

- Cecum and ascending colon (16%): Indigestion, weight loss, liquid stools, anemia, shortness of breath, weakness, dark red blood in stool, and dull abdominal and back pain.

Diagnosis

Diagnosis may begin with a barium enema or flexible sigmoidoscopy followed by colonoscopy if lesions are suspected higher in the large intestine. Endoscopic examination and biopsy are used to provide definitive proof of cancerous lesions. Laboratory studies such as carcinoembryonic antigen are useful as a prognostic tool and to evaluate the effectiveness of various treatments. Other diagnostic studies also may be helpful. The most important diagnostic tests include a complete blood count to evaluate for anemia; serum gamma-glutamyl transpeptidase, serum alkaline phosphatase, lactic dehydrogenase, serum glutamic oxaloacetic transaminase, and serum glutamic pyruvic transaminase to evaluate liver metastasis; and a chest radiograph, bone scan, liver scan, or computerized tomography scanning to identify the spread of the tumor to adjacent organs.

Staging

In the past, Duke's classification was the most widely used form of colon cancer staging. In more recent years, the tumor-node-metastasis staging is being used most often. See Table 7.1 for a comparison of the two staging classifications (Beart, 1991).

The metastasis pattern for colorectal cancer occurs by direct extension and penetration into the layers of the bowel followed by invasion to surrounding organs, into adjacent lymph nodes, and up the mesenteric lymph node chain. These tumors also have direct access to the vascular system once they have invaded the submucosa. Lymphatic disease occurs in 50% of cases. With extensive lymphatic spread, distant metastasis occurs in the liver and lungs and also may occur in the bone, brain, and adrenal glands. Cancer in the anal area invades directly into the muscles and genitourinary organs and can metastasize to the liver and lung.

Invasive and Noninvasive Management

Surgery

Surgical resection is the primary treatment option for 75% of cases. Radical resection is chosen most often because 70%–80% of rectal cancers present with direct extension or lym-

Table 7.1. Staging Classifications

Duke's Classification	T-N-M	Description
Duke's A	$T_1 N_0 M_0$	Limited to the mucosa
	$T_2 N_0 M_0$	Limited to the mucosa
Duke's B	$T_3 N_0 M_0$	Penetrates the serosa and connective tissue
	$T_4 N_0 M_0$	Invades other surrounding organs
Duke's C	any T $N_1 M_0$	Involved lymph nodes
	any T $N_2 M_0$	Involved lymph nodes
Duke's C2	any T $N_3 M_0$	Completely penetrates bowel wall
Duke's D	any T any N M_1	Any tumor with distant metastases

phatic spread (Parker et al., 1996). The type of surgery is determined by the location of the tumor. The major surgeries performed for colorectal cancers are

- Lower rectum (7 cm from anal verge): Abdominal perineal resection and colostomy
- Upper rectum (12 cm from anal verge): Pull through procedure
- Sigmoid colon (sigmoid portion of bowel): Sigmoid resection
- Left colon (splenic flexure and ascending colon): Colectomy or colostomy
- Right colon (cecum, ascending colon, proximal, and mid-transverse colon): Right colectomy or colostomy.

In many cases, the new bowel stapling devices have eliminated the need for a colostomy, except for those tumors that are in the rectum or near the anus (Renneker, 1988). Each case must be evaluated according to the individual patient's needs, taking into consideration the age, general physical health, nutritional status, and metastases. Gastrointestinal surgery in people over 80 years of age has been shown to have a high risk for complications and significantly more deaths. However, these procedures should not be denied because of age alone, especially if a curative operation is possible (Brocklehurst, Tallis, & Fillet, 1992).

A major responsibility of nursing care includes preoperative teaching. The patient should be prepared for the physiological and psychological changes throughout the perioperative period. When dealing with adults over age 70, the nurse must assess the patient's ability for self-care while assessing learning and psychomotor skill potential. Alterations in hearing, vision, and manual dexterity are essential elements to take into consideration prior to planning the nursing interventions as part of a nursing care plan that includes patient teaching (McConnell, 1988). Most older adults are capable of self-care, but involving family members in that care can be vitally important during the initial days after discharge from the hospital. Older adult patients need to be reassured that they will be able to become competent with ostomy care so that their independence can be preserved. An enterostomal nursing specialist can be most helpful with this specialized instruction. A typical teaching plan should include (Snyder, 1986)

- Location of the stoma
- Appearance of the stoma in the beginning (edematous) and later (smaller in six to eight weeks)
- Identification of appliances and application
- Importance of good skin care
- Type of fecal matter to expect from the specific stoma anticipated (colostomy—formed stool; ileostomy—constant liquid stool)
- Type of ostomy irrigation needed (colostomy requires irrigation; ileostomy is never irrigated)
- Instruction in proper diet to maintain good bowel functioning.

Chemotherapy

Administration of chemotherapy is effective as an adjunct therapy in colorectal cancer that is residual, advanced, or metastatic. Chemotherapy usually is used in combination with surgery or as a radiation sensitizer. The most widely used chemotherapy in this type of cancer and the side effects (Murphy, 1997) are

- 5-fluorouracil (5-FU) alone or in combination with methyl lomustine (MeCCNU, semustine). Side effects of 5-FU are anorexia, nausea, vomiting, stomatitis, diarrhea, bone marrow suppression, alopecia, dermatitis, and skin hyperpigmentation. If combined with MeCCNU, pulmonary fibrosis may occur.
- Levamisole plus 5-FU has been used after surgery to reduce disease recurrence and have proven beneficial in treating advanced disease (stage: Duke's C) to improve survival. Side effects are nausea, vomiting, fatigue, weakness, and dermatitis. Agranulocytosis and leuko-

penia have been observed in as many as 8% of patients with rheumatoid arthritis and cancer who were treated with this combination of drugs.

- Other drugs that are sometimes used in combination with 5-FU are mitomycin-C, methotrexate, cisplatin, vincristine, and leucovorin. However, 5-FU remains the drug of choice for treatment.

Patient and family teaching should include instructions on the potential side effects of drug therapy and advice on common remedies for ill effects. The major side effects of chemotherapy are presented along with recommended nursing interventions.

- **Nausea and vomiting** can cause excessive weight loss with fluid and electrolyte imbalance. This can occur very rapidly in older adults. Treatment with appropriate antiemetics before, during, and after therapy should be implemented, and responses should be monitored. Assessment for other causes of nausea and vomiting such as obstruction, constipation, pain, and effects of other medications should be included. Several types of antiemetics may be needed to control this symptom. The oral route may be used pretreatment. However, the rectal route may be necessary post-treatment. Antiemetics should be taken at least 30 minutes before meals for full effectiveness. Frequent small meals with adequate rest periods after meals and increased fluid intake should be encouraged. Rapid weight loss may cause a change in stoma size, which may require alteration in size or type of pouch used over the colostomy.
- **Diarrhea** is very common with 5-FU therapy and can be the first sign of severe toxicity. Diarrhea also is particularly distressing to the ostomy patient because skin breakdown occurs very easily, especially with older adults. Use of protective barriers to minimize contact of liquid stool with skin can assist in reducing the risk of skin rash and breakdown. Use of antidiarrheal agents may be needed if stools are passed too frequently. Liquid intake should be encouraged at 3,000 cc per day. This is needed to replace the additional lost fluids in stool. A diet low in residue but high in calories and proteins should be offered. Avoidance of foods and beverages containing caffeine needs to be reinforced.
- **Constipation** may occur and an assessment must be made to rule out bowel obstruction. This symptom may be a preexisting problem in older adults; therefore, a history of bowel habits is needed to compare current symptoms. Treatment includes moderate exercise, stool softeners, laxatives, and increased fluid intake.
- **Anorexia** is a major concern with this type of chemotherapy. The patient's weight needs to be monitored with each visit. A dietary history should be obtained, including food preferences, allergies, taste changes, and lactose intolerance. Medication for nausea and vomiting can be initiated if this is a problem. An appetite stimulant can be ordered along with nutritional supplements and an increase in high-protein foods such as milk, cheese, and yogurt. The patient education includes instructions on avoiding large quantities of fluids before meals, as this may cause feelings of fullness. Foods at room temperature usually are better tolerated, and exercise prior to meals will stimulate appetite (Otto, 1997).
- **Special precautions,** such as the use of a protective skin barrier around the stoma, may help to prevent bowel drainage from infused chemotherapy coming in contact with periostomal skin.
- **Fungal infection** occurs in the periostomal area from chemotherapy-induced bone marrow depression. Antifungal powders usually prove to be helpful.

Radiation

Adjuvant radiation therapy when combined with surgery has proven to be advantageous in reducing the incidence of local recurrence of colorectal cancer (Belcher, 1992). Radiation therapy can be administered pre- or postoperatively. The reasons for preoperative therapy (Hampton, 1993) are

- To improve the rate of surgical resectability
- To reduce the risk of spread of cancer cells locally or to distant sites during surgery
- To reduce the number of positive lymph nodes.

Surgery usually can proceed within two to three weeks after completion of radiation. The disadvantage of this type of treatment is that the histopathology of the tumor could be altered and, thus, compromise the comparison of treatment outcomes and staging (Hampton, 1993).

Postoperative radiation is used in high-risk patients to prevent recurrence. People who have tumors that have penetrated the bowel wall or who have positive lymph nodes are candidates for this treatment. Local recurrence of the tumor is decreased, but distant metastasis continues to remain a problem, and any alteration in survival rate is unclear (Rostock, Zajac, & Gallagher, 1992). Radiation therapy usually is started three to six weeks after surgery.

Using low doses of preoperative radiation and high doses of postoperative radiation has been beneficial. Tumor dissemination is decreased prior to surgery without compromising staging ability, and high-dose radiation then is used after surgery to treat those with pathologically confirmed advanced disease (Rostock et al., 1992).

The side effects of radiation to the abdominal and pelvic areas are diarrhea, nausea, bloating, fatigue, skin irritation, vaginal dryness, and cystitis. Teaching needs to include the importance of good nutrition, skin care, adequate rest, and potential alterations in sexuality. Eighty-five percent of patients receiving radiation to the bowel develop diarrhea, and the severity depends on the total dose of radiation, previous bowel habits, and lactose intolerance. Diarrhea usually occurs within two weeks of completion of therapy but may appear during treatment. In older adults, this side effect can be incapacitating, especially when coexisting medical problems have weakened the system and affected the appetite. If radiation occurs after surgery, the patient's nutritional status has been compromised because of the inability to ingest food during the postoperative period. Many older adult patients will be placed on hyperalimentation during this time to assist in maintaining the nutritional balance needed for healing.

Preradiation instructions include information on the expected length and frequency of treatments, how to care for skin markings, and preparations for potential side effects and management interventions. Physical care instructions must be supplemented with emotional support that may include discussion of coping mechanisms.

- **Diarrhea** is a common problem that usually occurs after treatment and is caused by the rapid proliferation of the epithelial cells in the intestinal wall. Antidiarrheal medications usually are effective. Rectal irritation often occurs and can be treated with creams or sitz baths. Ostomy patients may experience excoriation of the periostomal skin that may require the use of a skin barrier or the assistance of an enterostomal nursing specialist. If diarrhea occurs during treatment, radiation may need to be postponed until symptoms subside.
- **Nausea and vomiting** occur because of the destruction of the epithelial lining of the bowel wall. This cellular destruction creates a toxin that stimulates the nausea receptors in the brain. To prevent excessive weight loss and electrolyte imbalance, this must be controlled. The use of antiemetics several hours before treatment and continued use during the course of treatment will aid in preventing or decreasing the episodes of nausea and vomiting. Small frequent meals and liquid supplements will assist in maintaining nutritional status. Weight should be monitored weekly, and if a significant loss occurs, a more aggressive antiemetic regimen needs to be considered. Often several types of antiemetics need to be combined to control this symptom.
- **Sexual dysfunction** may occur in male and female patients. Men may have erectile and ejaculatory problems. Women may experience vaginal dryness and discomfort with intercourse. Several publications are available from the American Cancer Society that openly dis-

cuss these problems and suggest alternate forms of sexual contact, which may be very helpful to the patient and significant other.

- **Local skin irritation** from destruction of epithelial tissue can result in itching, dry skin areas, mild excoriation, and darkened areas at or near the radiation sites. Good skin cleansing with mild soap, warm water, and gentle patting to dry will help to avoid additional irritation to the area. Creams, lotions, and powders are not to be used unless prescribed by the radiation oncologist. The skin needs to be protected from extreme temperatures, so the use of heating pads or ice packs is not recommended. A light dusting with cornstarch is useful if pruritus occurs. Some individuals receive treatment with the use of parallel opposing portals, and only the portal on one side of the body may be marked. Check the skin on the opposing side and give it the same attention as the side with the markings (Hilderley, 1997).
- **Fatigue or malaise** is a common occurrence during and after treatment. Some helpful suggestions for patients are to get extra rest and reduce activities until energy levels return. A nap after treatment, going to bed earlier at night, and not attempting to fight the feelings of fatigue often are effective solutions. Fatigue may be greater in elderly patients, so instruct them to keep rest periods short during the day to prevent disturbing the nightly sleep pattern.

Special Problems

Bowel obstruction is the result of growing or recurring tumors. Tumors of the right colon usually do not result in obstruction for several reasons. Tumors in this area typically grow in, rather than around, the bowel. The tumors most often are large and bulky. However, the lumen of the ascending colon is much larger in diameter than other areas of the colon and can handle the increased bulk. A much larger mass can be present without compromising the bowel function. An important fact is that stool in this area of the bowel is liquid and can pass through a smaller opening. Obstruction is more likely in the transverse colon because of the narrowing of the bowel lumen, especially at the hepatic and splenic flexures, and the thickening consistency of stool.

The descending and sigmoid colon have varying degrees of obstruction as a result of the type of tumor usually found in the area. Annula or ring type tumors and scirrhous or solid hard tumors are common and cause a decrease in the size of the bowel lumen. This, in combination with the increased consistency of stool and decreased peristaltic action, contributes to the occurrence of obstructive episodes (Boarini, 1990).

Palliative Care

Patients with advanced malignant disease will benefit from palliative treatment. A number of treatment options now are available for patients with advanced cancer who develop intestinal obstruction.

Surgical treatment aimed at restoring the continuity of the bowel lumen always should be considered when bowel obstruction occurs. Many patients who undergo surgical resection, decompression, or bypass will enjoy a long and symptom-free period following palliative surgery.

Several factors must be considered when contemplating surgical intervention. These factors include age, general medical condition, and nutritional status. The presence of ascites or palpable masses or previous radiotherapy make successful surgery less likely (Baines, 1993).

The patient's wishes must be considered. Some patients will want to try every option that may prolong life. The very ill may choose symptomatic options. No patient should be coerced into surgery to prevent a distressing death from an obstruction because alternatives are available. These include the use of drugs that can prevent or control the symptoms.

The use of a nasogastric tube to decompress the stomach frequently is not effective over an extended time period and may require hospital admission. An alternative to the nasogastric tube is a venting gastrostomy tube to relieve vomiting. This can be placed by endoscope and does not require hospitalization. The need for home healthcare referral is paramount to ensure proper teaching and maintenance of the tube. Using this method, patients have been treated successfully and have survived comfortably for several months.

If surgery is considered inappropriate and long-term conservative treatment with a nasogastric tube or a venting gastrostomy tube does not relieve the patient's distress, pharmacologic management can be effective. Hospice care is very appropriate during this period to help manage the medications, support the family, and assist the patient in end-of-life issues. The course of treatment used during this time consists of controlling pain with the use of opioids, which are sufficient to relieve the pain but still allow the patient to be aware of his or her surroundings without extreme sedation. The use of corticosteroids, such as dexamethasone to reduce peri-tumor edema, may cause a reduction in the obstruction and a resultant relief of symptoms. Along with the steroids, the use of haloperidol 0.5–1.0 mg every 8–12 hours acts on the chemoreceptor trigger zone to reduce nausea and vomiting (Johanson, 1994).

Conclusion

The care that is provided to the patient and the teaching and support offered to the family or caregivers will be measured against expected outcomes established early in the course of nursing care. Among the outcome measures that the nurse anticipates are

- Recovery from any surgical procedure with stable intestinal functioning.
- Consistent ability to perform ostomy care with minimal assistance and discomfort.
- Effective coping patterns following the course of treatment through recovery.

With early diagnosis and treatment, the older adult with colorectal cancer can return to a satisfying quality of life. Early intervention can provide an operation intended for cure from this specific type of cancer.

References

American Cancer Society. (1996). Guidelines on diet, nutrition, and cancer prevention. *CA: A Cancer Journal for Clinicians, 46*, 325–341.

American Cancer Society. (1998). *Cancer facts and figures—1998.* Atlanta: Author.

Baines, M. (1993). The pathophysiology and management of malignant intestinal obstruction. In D. Doyle, G. Hanks, & N. MacDonald (Eds.), *Oxford textbook of palliative medicine* (pp. 311–399). New York: Oxford University Press.

Beart, R.W. (1991). Colorectal cancer. In A.I. Holleb, D.J. Fink, & G.P. Murphy (Eds.), *American Cancer Society textbook of clinical oncology* (pp. 213–218). Atlanta: American Cancer Society.

Belcher, A.E. (1992). Colorectal and other gastrointestinal cancers. In A. Belcher (Ed.), *Cancer nursing* (pp. 81–90). St. Louis: Mosby.

Boarini, J. (1990). Gastrointestinal cancer: Colon, rectum, and anus. In S.L. Groenwald, M.H. Frogge, M. Goodman, & C.H. Yarbro (Eds.), *Cancer nursing: Principles and practice* (2nd ed.) (pp. 702–805). Boston: Jones and Bartlett.

Brocklehurst, J.C., Tallis, R.C., & Fillit, H.M. (1992). The large bowel. In J.C. Brocklehurst, R.C. Tallis, & H.M. Fillit (Eds.), *Textbook of geriatric medicine and gerontology* (pp. 585–591). Edinburgh, Scotland: Churchill Livingstone.

Cohen, A.M., Minsky, B.D., & Schilsky, R.L. (1993). Colorectal cancer. In V.T. DeVita, S. Hellman, & S.A. Rosenberg (Eds.), *Cancer: Principles and practice of oncology* (4th ed.) (pp. 1144–1185). Philadelphia: Lippincott-Raven.

Giovannucci, E., Rimm, E.B., Ascherio, A., Stampfer, M.J., Colditz, G.A., & Willett, W.C. (1995). Alcohol, low-methionine—Low-folate diets and risk of colon cancer in men. *Journal of the National Cancer Institute, 87*, 265–273.

Hampton, B. (1993). Gastrointestinal cancer: Colon, rectum, and anus. In S.L. Groenwald, M.H. Frogge, M. Goodman, & C. Yarbro (Eds.), *Cancer nursing: Principles and practice* (3rd ed.) (pp. 1044–1064). Boston: Jones and Bartlett.

Hardcastle, J.D. (1997). Colorectal cancer. *CA: A Cancer Journal for Clinicians, 47*, 66–68.

Hilderley, L.J. (1997). Radiotherapy. In S. Groenwald, M. Frogge, M. Goodman, & C. Yarbro (Eds.), *Cancer nursing: Principles and practice* (4th ed.) (pp. 247–282). Boston: Jones and Bartlett.

Johanson, G.A. (1994). Bowel obstruction. In G.A. Johanson (Ed.), *Physicians handbook of symptom relief in terminal care* (pp. 14.1–14.3). Santa Rosa, CA: Sonoma County Academic Foundation for Excellence in Medicine.

McConnell, E.S. (1988). Nursing diagnosis related to physiological alteration. In M.A. Matteson & E.S. McConnell (Eds.), *Gerontological nursing concepts and practice* (pp. 331–427). Philadelphia: Saunders.

Murphy, M.E. (1997). Colorectal cancers. In S.E. Otto (Ed.), *Oncology nursing* (3rd ed.) (pp. 124–139). St. Louis: Mosby.

Otto, S.E. (Ed.). (1997). *Oncology nursing* (3rd ed.). St. Louis: Mosby.

Parker, S.L., Tong, T., Bolden, S., & Wingo, P.A. (1996). Cancer statistics, 1996. *CA: A Cancer Journal for Clinicians, 46*, 5–27.

Renneker, M. (1988). Cancer of the colon and rectum and anus. In M. Renneker (Ed.), *Understanding cancer* (pp. 136–138). Palo Alto, CA: Ball.

Rostock, R.A., Zajac, A.J., & Gallagher, M.J. (1992). Radiation therapy in the treatment of colorectal cancer. In J.D. Ahlgren & J.S. MacDonald (Eds.), *Gastrointestinal oncology* (pp. 359–381). Philadelphia: Lippincott.

Snyder, C.C. (1986). Nursing care of the surgical oncology client. In C.C. Snyder (Ed.), *Oncology nursing* (pp. 93–115). Boston: Little, Brown, & Co.

Chapter Eight

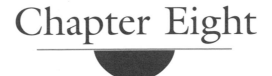

Treatment and Care of the Older Adult With Prostate Cancer

Ronda Kinsey, RN, MSN, AOCN®

Introduction

Prostate cancer is the most prevalent malignancy among American males, occurring in more than 184,000 men each year; nearly 40,000 men were expected to die from the disease in 1998 (Landis, Murray, Bolden, & Wingo, 1998). Men who have been diagnosed with prostate cancer face invasive diagnostic procedures, complex treatment decisions, and treatment morbidity that can affect every aspect of life. The physical and psychosocial effects of treatment are compounded by the fear of potential recurrence, progression, pain, and death.

Over the past decade, significant advances have been made in early detection, diagnosis, and treatment of prostate cancer. However, survival and quality-of-life issues continue to cause major concern for patients, families, and healthcare providers (Herr, 1997).

Epidemiology

Between 1976 and 1994, the incidence of prostate cancer doubled and mortality increased by 20%. Younger men were diagnosed with more localized disease than in previous time periods. These changes have been attributed to improvements in case findings rather than a true increase in disease prevalence. Prostate-specific antigen (PSA) screening and improvements in diagnostic methods (e.g., transrectal ultrasonography, biopsy technology) contributed to this progress. The annual incidence has stabilized since 1996 (Haas & Sakr, 1997).

Risk Factors

Age

Several factors are associated with an increased risk for development of prostate cancer, including age, family history, race, diet, and occupation. Prostate cancer primarily is a disease of older men. Rarely is it seen in men younger than age 50. However, age at diagnosis has decreased since the development of widespread prostate cancer screening. Before 1996, 62% of men diagnosed with prostate cancer each year were age 70 or older. Currently, only 53% of prostate cancer cases are diagnosed after age 70. As the aged population increases, prostate cancer is expected to become a growing health concern (Haas & Sakr, 1997).

Familial Patterns

Malignancies with familial patterns have been identified among men with prostate cancer. First-degree relatives (i.e., brothers or fathers) of men with the disease have a slightly higher risk of developing this malignancy. The risk increases in proportion to the number of affected relatives. Relatives of women with breast cancer also have a slightly higher risk for developing prostate cancer. Hereditary prostate cancer is characterized by early age of onset and is relatively uncommon, comprising only 9% of all cases (Haas & Sakr, 1997). Genetic testing for prostate cancer risk is available, but men are advised to seek genetic counseling prior to having the testing.

Race

African American men are at highest risk of developing and dying from this disease. The stage at diagnosis, socioeconomic factors, access to health services, and treatment selection factors may contribute to the high mortality rate (Haas & Sakr, 1997). However, some studies suggest that prognosis in this population is worse even with controls for stage, grade, and other clinical variables (Parker, Davis, Wingo, Ries, & Heath, 1998). Native Americans and Hispanic men have lower prostate cancer rates than other ethnic groups (Haas & Sakr).

Diet

Dietary differences may explain some of the variation in incidence of prostate cancer among different racial groups and geographic areas. For example, dietary fat has been implicated as a risk factor in some studies. High fat intake may cause alterations in hormonal levels that in some way support the development of prostate malignancy (Haas & Sakr, 1997).

Other Factors

Men employed in jobs that involve heavy physical labor or in rubber manufacturing and newspaper printing have a slightly higher incidence (Haas & Sakr, 1997). Men who reside in rural settings tend to present with later-stage disease. Studies of other potential risk factors (e.g., cigarette smoking, heavy metal exposure, sexual activity, sexually transmitted disease, vasectomy, benign prostatic hypertrophy [BPH]) have been inconclusive.

Screening

The American Cancer Society (ACS) recommends annual digital rectal examination (DRE) and PSA testing, beginning at age 50, for men with a life expectancy of 10 years or more (von Eschenbach, Ho, Murphy, Cunningham, & Lins, 1997). Younger men who have one or more relatives who have been diagnosed with prostate cancer also should be tested. Further evaluation should be considered if either test is abnormal. Although no studies currently demonstrate a direct effect on mortality rate, serial screening and appropriate treatment should prevent development of advanced prostate cancer, thereby decreasing the death rate from this disease (von Eschenbach et al.). The underlying assumption of the ACS recommendations is that early detection and treatment result in longer survival. This reasoning is consistent with a long-standing principle in oncology care. However, considerable controversy exists relative to the value of early detection and treatment of prostate cancer because, in some individuals, the treatment may be worse than the disease. In addition, costs of screening and early treatment may exceed the cost of late-stage treatment (Benoit & Naslund, 1997). Further research is needed to enable providers to predict with any certainty the cases likely to benefit from early treatment and to clarify the cost/benefit issues.

PSA

PSA is an enzyme that is produced in the epithelium of the prostate and periurethral glands. It aids in the liquefication of semen. A PSA level greater than 4.0 ng/ml generally is considered to be the threshold for biopsy. However, several other factors must be considered. Normal serum PSA levels increase with age. Several studies document age-specific reference ranges; however, the data published by Oesterling et al. (1993) currently are the standard.
- Age 40–49 years, 0.0–2.5 ng/ml
- Age 50–59 years, 0.0 3.5 ng/ml
- Age 60–69 years, 0.0–4.5 ng/ml
- Age 70–79 years, 0.0–6.5 ng/ml

PSA levels greater than 4.0 ng/ml are present in 25% of men with BPH. Also, 25% of men with prostate malignancy have PSA levels below 4.0 ng/ml (DeAntoni, 1997). PSA levels of 10 ng/ml or higher usually are indicative of malignancy (Trump, Shipley, Dillioglugil, & Scardino, 1997). Serial PSA testing is useful in monitoring disease progression in cases with elevated levels at the time of diagnosis; however, PSA tests are not reliable indicators of stage (DeAntoni).

Grade

Tumor grade is the most reliable indicator of prostate cancer behavior (Oesterling, Fuks, Lee, & Scher, 1997). Predicting the behavior of prostate cancer in a given individual is important. In some cases, the disease may never cause symptoms. In such circumstances, the treatment very well could be worse than the disease. In other cases, the disease may be very aggressive and destructive, and treatment can help to preserve both quantity and quality of life.

Several grading systems are described in the literature, although the Gleason system is the best known and most precise scale for predicting the behavior of the disease. The Gleason system identifies five levels of differentiation, or maturity, based on cellular architecture (see Figure 8.1). Because tissue specimens often contain elements of more than one level of differentiation, both primary and secondary architecture patterns are reported along with the sum (e.g., 2 + 5 = 7). Scores can range from 2 (e.g., 1 + 1 = 2) to 10 (e.g., 6 + 4 = 10). Lower scores indicate well-differentiated, more mature cellular structures and more indolent disease. Higher scores rep-

Figure 8.1. Histopathologic Grade and Gleason Score

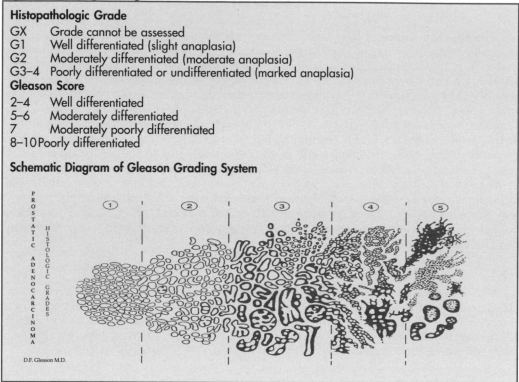

Histopathologic Grade

GX   Grade cannot be assessed
G1   Well differentiated (slight anaplasia)
G2   Moderately differentiated (moderate anaplasia)
G3–4   Poorly differentiated or undifferentiated (marked anaplasia)

Gleason Score

2–4   Well differentiated
5–6   Moderately differentiated
7   Moderately poorly differentiated
8–10 Poorly differentiated

Schematic Diagram of Gleason Grading System

D.F. Gleason M.D.

Note. Used with the permission of the American Joint Committee on Cancer (AJCC), Chicago, IL. The original source for this material is the *AJCC Manual for Staging of Cancer,* 5th edition (1997) published by Lippincott-Raven Publishers, Philadelphia.

resent more poorly differentiated cellular architecture and suggest more aggressive disease behavior. Correct interpretation of the Gleason score requires knowledge of both scores and sum, which is now considered feasible and reliable even when tissue samples are small, as with fine-needle aspiration biopsy specimens (Epstein, 1996).

Pathogenesis

Anatomy and Physiology

Discussion of prostate cancer pathophysiology will be aided by a brief review of normal anatomy and physiology. The normal prostate gland is approximately 4–6 centimeters in diameter and weighs approximately 20 grams. It is located beneath the urinary bladder and encircles the neck of the bladder and the urethra (Held-Warmkessel, 1997). In an embryo, the prostate contains five lobes (i.e., posterior, middle, anterior, and two lateral lobes). These become fused into three rather indistinct lobes during development (i.e., two lateral lobes on either side of the urethra and a smaller median lobe located at the floor of the urethra). The median lobe includes the embryonic posterior lobe, where most malignancies occur (Oesterling et al., 1997). Although references to a prostate capsule are common in clinical practice and in the literature, there is no distinct anatomical capsule surrounding the prostate gland. Such references are intended to distinguish organ-confined tumors from malignancies that extend into the surrounding soft tissue (Epstein, 1996).

The prostate gland produces 20% of the seminal fluid and other substances involved in sperm motility, but the gland is not essential to fertility. Secretory epithelial cells and stromal cells make up the two major tissue components of the prostate. The secretory epithelial cells contain androgen receptors. Androgen is required for their growth and for production of PSA and prostate-specific acid phosphatase (PAP). The stromal cells of the prostate produce 5 a-reductase, which converts androgens, primarily testosterone, to a-dihydrotestosterone (DHT). DHT binds with intracellular androgen receptors to trigger the segments of DNA that regulate the balance between cellular reproduction, differentiation, and death. In the absence of androgen, these cells die through a process called apoptosis (Oesterling et al., 1997).

Malignancy

Malignancy results when genetic changes occur in the regulatory segments of DNA and cells proliferate without the usual controls. Most prostate malignancies (99%) are adenocarcinoma (glandular). Other cell types include mucinous adenocarcinoma, small cell carcinoma, mixed small cell and adenocarcinoma, and prostatic duct adenocarcinomas. Each of these latter histologies portends aggressive disease, poor treatment response, and limited survival (Epstein, 1996).

Adenocarcinoma typically arises in the periphery of the prostate and spreads locally through the base of the bladder and seminal vesicles. The urethra and rectum also can become involved. Distant metastasis occurs via blood and lymphatic vessels and most often includes bone (i.e., spine, femur, pelvis, ribs, skull, and humerus, in order of frequency). The attraction of malignant prostate cells to bone is not fully understood, though one theory suggests a direct biochemical interaction between prostate epithelial cells and bone stroma. Bone metastases usually consist of osteoblastic and osteolytic components but primarily are osteoblastic. Prostate cancer also commonly spreads to the lungs, liver, and epidural space. Metastatic lesions usually are of the same histology as the primary site but sometimes contain the higher grade Gleason score of smaller secondary sites within the prostate when multi-focal lesions are present (Epstein, 1996).

Diagnosis

In the presence of an abnormal DRE or PSA, or progressive urinary symptoms, biopsy is recommended. Biopsy can be performed in an ambulatory setting through use of transrectal ultrasound guidance. A large-core needle triggered by a biopsy gun is used to obtain multiple samples from the abnormal area visualized on ultrasound and from each side of the prostate. Tissue specimens from the transition zone also may be sampled if clinically indicated. Fine-needle aspiration may be used as an alternative in some clinics (Oesterling et al., 1997).

Staging

The initiation of mass prostate cancer screening in the early 1980s resulted in diagnosis of the disease in its earliest stages. Both clinical and pathologic (i.e., tumor, nodes, metastases) staging systems are commonly used (see Figure 8.2). The extent of staging workup and the use of one or both staging systems depends on the individual situation. Because of the indolent

Figure 8.2. Primary Tumor (T or PT), Regional Lymph Nodes (N), Distant Metastasis (M) (TNM) Staging System

Primary Tumor and Clinical Stage

T_X	Primary tumor cannot be assessed.
T_0	No evidence of primary tumor exists.
T_1	Clinically inapparent tumor is not palpable nor visible by imaging.
T_{1a}	Tumor incidental histologic finding in 5% or less of tissue resected
T_{1b}	Tumor incidental histologic finding in more than 5% of tissue resected
T_{1c}	Tumor is identified by needle biopsy (e.g., because of elevated PSA).
T_2	Tumor is confined within prostate.*
T_{2a}	Tumor involves one lobe.
T_{2b}	Tumor involves both lobes.
T_3	Tumor extends through the prostate.**
T_{3a}	Extracapsular extension (unilateral or bilateral)
T_{3b}	Tumor invades seminal vesicles(s).
T_4	Tumor is fixed or invades adjacent structures other than seminal vesicles: bladder neck, external sphincter, rectum, levator muscles, and/or pelvic wall.

Primary Tumor and Pathologic Stage

PT_2***	Organ confined
PT_{2a}	Unilateral
PT_{2b}	Bilateral
PT_3	Extraprostatic extension
PT_{3a}	Extraprostatic extension
PT_{3b}	Seminal vesicle invasion
PT_4	Invasion of bladder and/or rectum

Regional Lymph Nodes (N)

N_X	Regional lymph nodes cannot be assessed.
N_0	No regional lymph node metastasis
N_1	Metastasis in regional lymph node or nodes

Distant Metastasis**** (M)

M_X	Distant metastasis cannot be assessed.
M_0	No distant metastasis
M_1	Distant metastasis
M_{1a}	Nonregional lymph node(s)
M_{1b}	Bone(s)
M_{1c}	Other site(s)

* Tumor found in one or both lobes by needle biopsy, but not palpable or reliably visible by imaging, is classified as $T1_c$.
** Invasion into the prostatic apex or into (but not beyond) the prostatic capsule is not classified as T_3, but as T_2.
*** There is no pathologic T_1 classification.
**** When more than one site of metastasis is present, the most advanced category is used. PM_{1c} is most advanced.

Note. Used with the permission of the American Joint Committee on Cancer (AJCC), Chicago, IL. The original source for this material is the *AJCC Manual for Staging of Cancer,* 5th edition (1997) published by Lippincott-Raven Publishers, Philadelphia.

nature of most prostate malignancies in elderly men, National Comprehensive Cancer Network (NCCN) guidelines recommend assessment of comorbidity and life expectancy before completing a full staging evaluation. If life expectancy is less than five years and no symptoms are present, no further workup should be performed. In fact, screening for asymptomatic disease is considered to be inappropriate if life expectancy is less than five years. When life expectancy is greater than five years, clinical staging is recommended, including a compete blood count (CBC) and PAP test. A bone scan is recommended only when the clinical stage is T_1 or T_2 with a PSA greater than 10 ng/ml, when the Gleason score is greater than 8, when the clinical stage is T_3 or T_4, or if the man reports bone pain. Computerized tomography (CT) scan or magnetic resonance imaging (MRI) may be warranted in individuals with disease staged at T_3 or T_4. Fine-needle aspiration is indicated if either of these tests reveal evidence of lymph node involvement (Oesterling et al., 1997).

Treatment

Although prostate cancer generally is considered to be a slow-growing disease, it can progress and become more problematic over time. Early disease usually is asymptomatic. Symptoms of advanced disease include bladder outlet obstruction (e.g., slow urinary stream, hesitancy, incomplete emptying, frequency, nocturia, dysuria). These symptoms also occur in the presence of BPH, but symptoms that become progressively worse usually indicate malignancy. If left untreated, total obstruction of the upper urinary tract or large bowel can occur. As the disease progresses, other symptoms may develop, including bone pain, pathologic fractures, hepatomegaly, edema of the lower extremities caused by enlarged pelvic lymph nodes, and mental confusion caused by central nervous system metastasis (Oesterling et al., 1997).

Treatment modalities for prostate cancer include radical prostatectomy, resection of the prostate gland, external-beam radiation, interstitial radioactive seed implantation, hormonal therapy, and watchful waiting. Treatment decisions hinge on prediction of which cases will cause significant problems in the individual's lifetime. Treatment selection must incorporate consideration of individual factors (e.g., age and general health) and disease-related factors (e.g., PSA levels, tumor volume, stage, Gleason score). In other words, an attempt must be made to predict the likelihood of the individual living long enough to suffer from the disease. In addition, the individual's personal preferences about the relative risks of the disease and potential treatment morbidity must be considered (Oesterling et al., 1997).

Treatment for organ-confined prostate cancer (i.e., T_1 and T_2, N_0) is controversial. NCCN recommends radical prostatectomy or radiation therapy. Expectant therapy (i.e., watchful waiting) also is a reasonable consideration in some cases. Multimodal therapy may be appropriate when the probability of relapse is high. Further research is needed to determine best practice (Millikan & Logothetis, 1997).

Locally advanced disease (i.e., clinical stages T_3 and T_4) should be treated with radiation therapy with or without total androgen ablation. Outcomes are better with these regimens than with radical prostatectomy (Millikan & Logothetis, 1997).

Advanced disease may be treated with radiotherapy or androgen ablation. Supportive therapies may include prednisone, spot radiation or radionuclide therapy for control of bone pain, and chemotherapy (Millikan & Logothetis, 1997; Oesterling et al., 1997).

Alternative and complementary therapies have become very popular for a variety of health problems. Alternative medicine is defined as "approaches to medical diagnosis and therapy that have not been developed by use of generally accepted scientific methods" (Thomas, 1997, p. 71). When these treatments are used in conjunction with standard methods, they are considered to be complementary. Strategies such as therapeutic touch, acupuncture, acupressure, massage, aromatherapy, guided imagery, biofeedback, reflexology, and herbal therapies can be used as alternative or complementary therapies. Their popularity necessitates that nurses become familiar with them and provide appropriate patient education to ensure safety. It is beyond the scope of this chapter to elaborate on all potential therapies, but two herbal preparations are of particular relevance to the care of men with prostate disease. Nettles and saw palmetto are sold as pharmaceuticals in Europe but are restricted by the U.S. Food and Drug Administration. They are, however, readily available as nutritional supplements in the United States.

Nettles and saw palmetto have been studied and approved in European countries for use in the treatment of prostate ailments. Nettles, or stinging nettles, are perennial plants found throughout the United States, Canada, and Europe. Tiny hairs on mature nettle leaves cause stinging and irritation to exposed skin. The leaves, which contain more than 24 chemicals, have been shown in German studies to increase urine output, decrease frequency of urination, and improve bladder emptying (Facts and Comparisons, 1997). The exact mechanism of action is not fully understood. One theory is that it reduces male hormone binding to cellular receptor sites. Side effects include contact urticaria and, rarely, other allergic responses. Claims that nettle is useful in the treatment of cancer, diabetes, rheumatoid arthritis, hair loss, and skin and scalp disorders lack substantive research (Facts and Comparisons, 1997).

Saw palmetto is a large palm that grows in southern areas of the United States. Saw palmetto berry teas and extracts have been used for many years as sexual stimulants. Oral absorption in tea or extract form is poor, and its value as an aphrodisiac is questionable. Research suggests that lipid fraction berry extracts may be useful in managing the nocturia, dysuria, and other symptoms of BPH. The potential benefits for BPH are derived through antiandrogenic effects on estrogen receptors and inhibition of an enzyme, testosterone-5-α-reductase, and by preventing conversion of testosterone to DHT. DHT binding at receptor sites also may be inhibited. Side effects, which include headache and diarrhea, are uncommon. Additional research is needed to clarify the value of saw palmetto extract in the treatment of BPH. Very little research exists on the use of saw palmetto in the treatment of prostate malignancy, and the potential hormonal effects contraindicate its use pending further study (Facts and Comparisons, 1994).

People who have been diagnosed with cancer are vulnerable and often receptive to treatment ideas from many sources. Nurses must be alert to the possibility that patients may self-treat prostate symptoms with alternative and complementary therapies without reporting their use to their healthcare providers unless questioned specifically about them. A nonjudgmental approach is essential. When herbal therapy use is discovered, collaboration with a clinical pharmacist who is familiar with the current research on herbal preparations may be advisable. Patients should be offered accurate, research-based information and encouraged to report alternative and complementary therapies to their primary healthcare provider, urologist, or medical oncologist.

Survival

With appropriate treatment, the five-year survival rate for localized prostate cancer is approximately 94%. Overall five-year survival for all stages is 80%. However, life expectancy with advanced prostate cancer is approximately one to two years (Oesterling et al., 1997).

Nursing Diagnoses and Plan of Care

Nursing diagnoses for patients with prostate cancer depend on many factors, including stage of disease, preexisting health problems, and individual response to treatment and rehabilitation. Impaired adjustment, anxiety, ineffective individual or family coping, altered sleep patterns, pain, fatigue, impaired home maintenance, and impaired mobility are diagnoses commonly associated with prostate malignancy in various stages of the disease. Nurses should be alert for evidence of these problems and intervene according to oncology and gerontology nursing standards. Four nursing diagnoses present challenges specific to the person with prostate cancer; these will be addressed in more detail.

Knowledge Deficit

The North American Nursing Diagnosis Association (NANDA) defined knowledge deficit as "an absence or deficiency of cognitive information or the inability to state or explain information or demonstrate a required skill. It is also the inability to explain or use self-care practices recommended to restore health or maintain wellness. It may present as a cognitive or psychomotor deficit or as a combination of the two" (McFarland & McFarlane, 1996, p. 502). The characteristics of this diagnosis (McFarland & McFarlane) include
- Verbalization of inadequate information or inadequate recall of information
- Verbalization of misunderstanding or misconception
- Requesting information; instructions inaccurately followed
- Inadequate performance on a test
- Inadequate demonstration of a skill

In the context of providing nursing care for men with prostate cancer, knowledge deficits should be anticipated and systematically assessed. Knowledge deficits may be related to procedures, treatment options, potential side effects, role functions, or managing incontinence, to name only a few. A recent study revealed that men with prostate cancer are most interested in learning about the disease process, chances for cure, and types of treatment available (Davison, Degner, & Morgan, 1995). However, each individual should be assessed and priority should be given to the information about which he is most concerned. Additional information that is necessary for self-care and healthy adjustment should be offered after the individual's priority concerns are addressed.

Each individual's learning readiness, education level, cognitive abilities, and culture should be considered. For example, attention deficits caused by the stress of the illness, medications, and preexisting memory problems may impede understanding. Cultural or language differences also must be considered. Teaching methods should be selected according to individual needs and may include individual or group instruction and the use of written, audio, or video media. Written materials are available from the National Cancer Institute and ACS (O'Rourke & Germino, 1998). Patients and family members often seek advice from nonprofessionals, including family and friends, and may need assistance in sorting out pertinent facts from well-intended misinformation.

Decisional Conflict

Decisional conflict is defined as "the uncertainty about which course of action to take when choice among competing actions involves risk, loss, regret, or challenge to personal life values" (McFarland & McFarlane, 1996, p. 486). Difficulties in decision making often are apparent in the verbalized concerns of patients. Nonverbal cues such as muscle tension, restlessness, and increased heart rate also should be assessed and validated. For men with prostate cancer, the focus of a decisional conflict may be the choice between radical prostatectomy and radiation therapy, whether to discuss embarrassing and very private distress about impotence openly with the urologist, or how to tell family members about advancing disease. The sources of decisional conflict are as varied as the number of men facing this disease each year.

Regardless of the issue, expectations and personal values factor heavily into the decision-making process. Misconceptions about radiation therapy and surgery can interfere with decision making (O'Rourke & Germino, 1998). Nursing assessment of each of these aspects is, therefore, an essential first step in assisting a patient into action.

- What does the individual expect as the outcome of each choice?
- Does he have an accurate understanding of each treatment?
- What is the meaning or significance of each choice and each outcome to the patient?
- Which option is most tolerable?
- Which option is least tolerable?

Another important factor is the patient's decision-making preference. While some individuals may prefer to make treatment decisions independently, others prefer to share the responsibility with their physicians. Many people, especially older adults, want their physicians to make the final decision. Decision-making preferences should be assessed and communicated to physicians and others involved in the treatment decision process (Davison et al., 1995).

Altered Urinary Elimination: Incontinence

NANDA defined altered urinary elimination as "the state in which an individual experiences a disturbance in urine elimination" (McFarland & McFarlane, 1996, p. 261). Urinary retention and incontinence are possible after prostate cancer treatment. Radical prostatectomy results in temporary urinary incontinence for most men in the immediate postoperative period. However, 12–24 months after surgery, 8%–45% of men experience some degree of persistent incontinence (Oesterling et al., 1997). The incidence varies among the studies published and with the type of surgical procedure performed. External-beam radiotherapy rarely causes incontinence, and fewer than 0.5% of men report incontinence after radioactive seed implant when those individuals have not had previous transurethral resection of the prostate (TURP) (Roddy et al., 1997). However, urinary incontinence is fairly common (48%) after interstitial seed implant among men with a previous TURP (Roddy et al.). Symptoms of chronic cystitis occur in approximately 13% of men after external-beam therapy (Oesterling et al., 1997) and in 3%–7% after radioactive seed implant therapy (Roddy et al.).

The physiologic mechanism causing incontinence probably involves damage to the sphincter, causing sphincter insufficiency and stress incontinence (i.e., involuntary urination with coughing or sneezing) or bladder dysfunction resulting in urge incontinence (i.e., bladder contractions occurring with the urge to urinate) (Harris, 1997).

Preexisting urinary function problems may confound the effects of prostate cancer treatment as with chronic conditions (e.g., alcoholism, Alzheimer's disease, diabetes mellitus, Parkinson's disease, cerebral vascular accident) and acute problems (e.g., fecal impaction and constipation, medication effects such as diuretics, age-related changes such as decreased capacity, incomplete emptying, contractions during filling, retention of residual urine).

The psychosocial consequences of urinary incontinence can be devastating for the individual and his caregiver or partner. The embarrassment of uncontrolled urination can lead to self-imposed social isolation, work role changes, and depression (Chiverton, Wells, Brink, & Mayer, 1996). To assist the patient in learning to manage and cope with urinary incontinence, a thorough assessment of all contributing factors is essential. Assessment should include usual 24-hour fluid intake, frequency of urination, frequency of incontinence, nocturia, dysuria, precipitating factors (e.g., cough, changing positions), sensory cues, and ability to start and stop the urinary stream (Pearson & Kelber, 1996).

Nurses should consider potential environmental adjustments, physiologic and behavioral methods, and containment options when planning interventions.

- Environmental adjustments, such as placing a urinal near the bed at night and removing obstacles in the path to the bathroom, may be helpful.
- Behavioral methods may include smoking cessation to reduce cough, increased fluid intake, regular toileting, pelvic floor muscle exercises, and constipation prevention (Harris, 1997; Pearson & Kelber, 1996).
- Physiologic intervention options may include medications (e.g., alpha adrenergics or anticholinergics) and sphincter reconstruction (Roddy et al., 1997).
- Containment should be considered a temporary intervention pending improvement in urinary function through other methods. External catheters and disposable pads may be helpful adjuncts to other therapies until continence can be achieved.

Sexual Dysfunction: Impotence

NANDA defined sexual dysfunction as "the state in which problems with sexual function exist" (McFarland & McFarlane, 1996, p. 777). This definition encompasses changes in sexual desire, arousal, and orgasm associated with physical or psychological illness. Sexual function is associated with depression (Araujo, Durante, Feldman, Goldstein, & McKinlay, 1998) and is an important predictor of quality of life after prostate cancer (Herr, 1997).

Sexual dysfunction is common after treatment for prostate cancer because of disruption of the autonomic nerve pathways in the pelvis. Impotence, or erectile dysfunction, develops in 39%–70% of men within one to five years after receiving external-beam irradiation (Oesterling et al., 1997). After interstitial radioactive seed implant, 20%–25% of men older than age 70 with normal preoperative erectile function will become impotent within the first one to two years. The incidence is lower (10%–15%) for younger men (Roddy et al., 1997). Temporary impotence occurs in all men immediately after radical prostatectomy and gradually improves over time for some. Thirty-one percent to 85% of men are impotent for one to two years after surgery. Men who achieve erection after surgical removal of the prostate gland experience retrograde ejaculation into the bladder because of the reduced backflow resistance. Although these men retain sexual functions of erection and experience orgasmic pleasure, the reduction of ejaculant may be misinterpreted if not explained prior to surgery.

Treatment options for erectile dysfunction include external ischiocavernous muscle stimulation, penile prosthesis, and medications (e.g., alpha blockers, Viagra® [Pfizer Inc., New York, NY]). Nurses, recognizing that sexuality is a very private concern for older adults, can influence quality of life by asking about sexual function as part of the routine patient assessment, educating men about the risk of impotence associated with prostate cancer treatment, and providing information about erectile dysfunction treatment.

Conclusion

Nurses have an important role in the care and treatment of men with prostate cancer. Nurses, more than any other healthcare provider, are prepared to recognize the unique characteristics of aging that may influence learning, decision making, self-care, and recovery. The ability to integrate that information for effective interventions is a major goal of nursing care.

References

Araujo, A.B., Durante, R., Feldman, H.A., Goldstein, I., & McKinlay, J.B. (1998). The relationship between depressive symptoms and male erectile dysfunction: Cross-sectional results from the Massachusetts male aging study. *Psychosomatic Medicine, 60,* 458–465.

Benoit, R.M., & Naslund, M.J. (1997). The economics of prostate cancer screening. *Oncology, 11,* 1533–1543.

Chiverton, P.A., Wells, T.J., Brink, C.A., & Mayer, R. (1996). Psychological factors associated with urinary incontinence. *CNS: The Journal for Advanced Nursing Practice, 10,* 229–233.

Davison, P.J., Degner, L.F., & Morgan, T.R. (1995). Information and decision-making preferences of men with prostate cancer. *Oncology Nursing Forum, 22,* 1401–1408.

DeAntoni, E.P. (1997). Age-specific reference ranges for PSA in the detection of prostate cancer. *Oncology, 11,* 475–485.

Epstein, J.I. (1996). Pathologic evaluation of prostatic carcinoma: Critical information for the oncologist. *Oncology, 10,* 527–534.

Facts and Comparisons. (1994, March). *Lawrence review of natural products: Saw palmetto.* St. Louis: Wolters Kluwer Co.

Facts and Comparisons. (1997, April). *Lawrence review of natural products: Nettles.* St. Louis: Wolters Kluwer Co.

Haas, G.P., & Sakr, W. (1997). Epidemiology of prostate cancer. *CA: A Cancer Journal for Clinicians, 47,* 273–287.

Harris, J.L. (1997). Treatment of post-prostatectomy urinary incontinence with behavioral methods. *CNS: The Journal for Advanced Nursing Practice, 11,* 159–166.

Held-Warmkessel, J. (1997). Prostate cancer. In S.L. Groenwald, M.H. Frogge, M. Goodman, & C.H. Yarbro (Eds.), *Cancer nursing: Principles and practice* (4th ed.) (pp. 1334–1354). Boston: Jones and Bartlett.

Herr, H.W. (1997). Quality of life in prostate cancer patients. *CA: A Cancer Journal for Clinicians, 47,* 207–217.

Landis, S.H., Murray, T., Bolden, S., & Wingo, P.A. (1998). Cancer statistics, 1998. *CA: A Cancer Journal for Clinicians, 48,* 6–30.

McFarland, G.K., & McFarlane, E.A. (Eds.). (1996). *Nursing diagnosis & intervention: Planning for patient care* (3rd ed.). St. Louis: Mosby.

Millikan, R., & Logothetis, C. (1997). Update of the NCCN guidelines for treatment of prostate cancer. *Oncology, 11,* 180–193.

Oesterling, J., Fuks, Z., Lee, C.T., & Scher, H.I. (1997). Cancer of the prostate. In V.T. DeVita, S.A. Rosenberg, & S. Hellman (Eds.), *Cancer: Principles and practice of oncology* (5th ed.) (pp. 1322–1386). Philadelphia: Lippincott-Raven.

Oesterling, J., Jacobsen, S.J., Chute, C.G., Guess, H.A., Girman, C.J., Panser, L.A., & Lieber, M.M. (1993). Serum prostate-specific antigen in a community-based population of healthy men: Establishment of age-specific reference ranges. *JAMA, 270,* 860–864.

O'Rourke, M.E., & Germino, B.B. (1998). Prostate cancer treatment decisions: A focus group exploration. *Oncology Nursing Forum, 25,* 97–104.

Parker, S.L., Davis, K.J., Wingo, P.A., Ries, A.G., & Heath, C.W. (1998). Cancer statistics by race and ethnicity. *CA: A Cancer Journal for Clinicians, 48,* 31–48.

Pearson, B.D., & Kelber, S. (1996). Urinary incontinence: Treatments, interventions, and outcomes. *CNS: The Journal for Advanced Nursing Practice, 10,* 177–182.

Roddy, T., Grimm, P.D., Ireton, R., Stull, P., Sylvester, J., & Downey, J. (1997). *Complications of permanent seed implantation.* Seattle: Northwest Prostate Institute, Swedish Medical Center.

Thomas, C.L. (Ed.). (1997). *Taber's® cyclopedic medical dictionary* (18th ed.). Philadelphia: F.A. Davis.

Trump, D.L., Shipley, W.U., Dillioglugil, O., & Scardino, P.T. (1997). Neoplasms of the prostate. In J.F. Holland, R.C. Bast, Jr., D.L. Morton, E. Frei, III, D.W. Kufe, & R.R. Weichselbaum (Eds.), *Cancer medicine* (4th ed.) (pp. 2125–2164). Philadelphia: Williams & Wilkins.

von Eschenbach, A., Ho, R., Murphy, G.P., Cunningham, M., & Lins, N. (1997). American Cancer Society guidelines for the early detection of prostate cancer: Update 1997. *CA: A Cancer Journal for Clinicians, 47,* 261–264.

Chapter Nine

Cancer Pain in the Older Adult

Ann Schmidt Luggen, PhD, RN, CS, CNAA, ARNP

Prevalence of Cancer Pain in Older Adults

Estimates of cancer pain in older adults are based upon cancer incidence (see Chapter 1) and pain prevalence data. Some information about pain in older adults is available, but few pain research studies have been conducted in this population, and fewer still have focused on cancer pain.

In one study, older adults with advanced cancer in a hospice setting were assessed for pain upon admission (Stein & Miech, 1993). Seventy-five percent of these patients reported pain. Stein (1996) observed that unrelieved pain not only destroys the quality of life in the final days of life but also leaves family members with tragic memories of their loved ones in those final days. In another hospice study, 33% of elderly patients reported significant pain, and 25% reported their worst pain just days before death (Morris et al., 1986).

Pain

The data available suggest that, in general, pain is a significant problem in elderly people (Brattberg, Parker, & Thorslund, 1996; Crook, Rideout, & Browne, 1984; Roy & Thomas, 1987; Stein & Ferrell, 1996; Sternbach, 1986). It is a problem even before retirement and is greater in older age groups (Bowsher, Rigge, & Sopp, 1991), specifically pain in the joints (Sternbach).

Among nursing home residents, pain appears to be a considerable problem (Bernabei et al., 1998). Pain prevalence in this population is estimated at 45%–80% (Ferrell, Ferrell, & Osterweil, 1990). Ferrell et al. (1990) reported that 71% of residents had at least one pain problem, and 34% described continuous pain; 66% described intermittent pain, and 51% described daily pain. Only 15% of these residents had received any pain medication in the previous 24 hours (Ferrell et al., 1990). In a recent study of nursing home residents with cancer conducted by Bernabei et al., only 26% of the patients received morphine, and those 85 and older were much less likely to receive morphine compared to those ages 65–74. More than 25% of residents received no analgesia at all. Horgas and Tsai (1998) reported that significantly fewer analgesics were prescribed and given (in number and in dose) to cognitively impaired residents in a long-term care setting. Physicians prescribed fewer analgesics, and nursing staff administered less.

Cancer Pain

The World Health Organization (WHO, 1990) estimated that approximately 75% of all patients with cancer will experience pain during their illness. Ventafridda, Tamburini, Caraceni, DeConno, and Naldi (1987) estimated pain to be a major symptom in at least 70% of patients with cancer. The incidence of cancer increases with age, so one may assume that a great deal of cancer pain is present in older adults with cancer (Stein & Miech, 1993).

Effects of Pain

In addition to the shock, denial, anxiety, and grief that occurs in almost any patient who receives a cancer diagnosis, pain, in older patients specifically, impairs social activities, mobility, sleep, bowel functions, and appetite and causes depression and anxiety (Stein & Ferrell, 1996). Other consequences of unrelieved cancer pain in older adults include fear, diminished quality of life, falls, polypharmacy, malnutrition, increased utilization of healthcare resources, increased healthcare costs, diminished progress in rehabilitation, cognitive dysfunction, and loss of hope (Stein, 1997).

Patients whose pain is related to diagnosis or treatment or occurs during the acute phase of a cancer diagnosis tend to remain hopeful and may endure pain without seeking relief with pain medications. Chronic cancer-related pain associated with progression of disease may cause feelings of hopelessness or helplessness to predominate (Foley, 1985).

Sleep disturbances are common in older adults. Cancer pain, especially related to bone metastases, may exacerbate this problem by causing constant pain, which often is worse at night or with movement (Patt, 1993a).

Pain Physiology and Aging

Older adults have many refractory nonmalignant chronic illnesses that cause pain (e.g., arthritis, osteoporosis, herpes zoster, trigeminal neuralgia, chronic back pain). Few studies of pain perception in older adults have been conducted, and age-related changes in pain receptors (presbyalgos) have not been established (Kelly & Payne, 1993). Some data suggest that older adults have higher pain reaction thresholds and lower pain tolerance (Harkins, Kwentus, & Price, 1990).

Pain is electrically transmitted after activation of nociceptors (pain receptors) by way of impulses along afferent nerve fibers. The A-delta fiber is "fast pain" and localized, producing a stinging or pricking sensation. C fibers are "slow," longer-lasting, generalized, and dull-aching in nature. One research report suggested that older adults rely on C-fiber input more than young people, who utilize additional input from A-delta fibers (Chakour, Gibson, Bradbeer, & Helme, 1996).

Cancer Pain Mechanisms

Cancer pain can be caused by the tumor, cancer treatment, or unrelated pain. Tumor invasion can be mechanical (causing pressure on other organs) and neurohumoral (causing compression or injury to peripheral nerves and/or to central nervous system) or be the result of sensitization of nerves to the effects of tumor pressure on normal tissues (Johnson & Parris, 1997).

Bone Pain

Bone pain is caused by tumor invasion of bone periosteum invoking an inflammatory response. Bone metastases are clinically evident in one-third of patients with cancer and found in two-thirds at autopsy (Foley, 1985). Pathological fractures cause significant pain in patients with cancer, especially in axial spine metastases (Johnson & Parris, 1997). Trauma to periosteum, peripheral nerve compression, or spinal cord compression is the pain mechanism. This occurs in cancers of the lung and breast and in lymphomas. Joint pain is a response to the inflammatory process provoked by the malignant process (Johnson & Parris).

Neurogenic Pain

This pain is caused by disruption of nerve axons by compression or infiltration of tumor. The expanding tumor mass can cause edema, ischemia, and necrosis, with resultant degeneration of axons and myelin sheaths. Compression of intracranial vessels from edema can cause pain. Neurogenic pain syndromes are very resistant to treatment (Johnson & Parris, 1997).

Peripheral Neuropathies

Neuropathies such as brachial plexopathy can result from breast and lung cancer invasion. Pain often is the presenting symptom (Johnson & Parris, 1997) and occurs in nearly 85% of patients with invasion of the brachial plexus from breast cancer (Patt, 1993a). It presents as a moderately severe ache of the shoulder radiating along the ulnar nerve. Movement of the upper extremity aggravates it.

Lumbosacral plexopathy can result from breast or colorectal cancer involving the pelvic wall with resultant pain in the anteromedial or anterolateral thigh. Following pain are symptoms of numbness and weakness (Johnson & Parris, 1997). In lumbosacral plexopathy, pain may be a valued external diagnostic sign. It was the presenting symptom in 70% of patients in one major study and was the only symptom in 24% of patients (Patt, 1993a).

Visceral Pain

Visceral pain is caused by infiltration, traction, or compression of hollow visceral outlets (e.g., bladder, intestine, stomach, uterus). Contraction and distention cause pain that is poorly localized, often referred to dermatomes supplied by spinal segments. Therefore, prostate infiltration may cause pain in the abdomen or leg; liver pain refers to the right shoulder; and endometrial pain refers to the back, in the paraspinal muscles (Johnson & Parris, 1997).

Vascular space infiltration may produce pain from venous engorgement, tissue edema, ischemia, lymphangitis, and peripheral nerve distribution. Breast cancer may cause edema of the upper extremity from axillary lymphadenopathy and edema of the lower extremity from obstruction of vascular structures by pelvic lymphadenopathy (Johnson & Parris, 1997).

Phantom Limb Pain

Phantom limb pain occurs in nearly 70% of amputees and often is intractable (Melzack, 1992). Patients have the sensation that the limb is real and may try to use the limb (e.g., lift a cup with a phantom hand). The pain is described as burning, cramping, or shooting in nature.

It can be occasional and mild or continuous and severe. It can start immediately after the amputation or years later. Eliminating PLP is very difficult (Melzack, 1992).

Paraneoplastic Pain Syndromes

Paraneoplastic pain syndromes (PPS) can accompany cancer. Common cancers of older adults associated with PPS are bronchogenic, breast, and prostate cancers. Some of the PPS include dermatomyositis, myopathy, and polymyositis, which cause a myalgic pain. Arthralgias and myalgias may be caused by rheumatoid arthritis or polymyalgia rheumatica (Johnson & Parris, 1997) or as a side effect of some chemotherapy treatments, especially the taxanes.

Chronicity

Cancer pain also may be classified as acute or chronic. Acute pain is associated with sympathetic hyperactivity and distress (Patt, 1993a). Acute pain occurs with procedures such as lumbar puncture, thoracentesis, and bone marrow biopsy. Chronic pain is more difficult to assess and manage. It actually may take on the status of a disease (Patt, 1993a) and contribute markedly to the patient's deterioration.

Common Sites of Nonmalignant Pain in Older Adults

Pain is very prevalent in older adults. Musculoskeletal problems such as osteoarthritis (OA), rheumatoid arthritis (RA), osteoporosis, and fractures affect more elderly people than any other chronic diseases. Common sites of these disorders include (Hewitt & Foley, 1996)
- Joints—Shoulders, hips, knees, and hands (OA, RA)
- Spine—Lumbar disk stenosis (OA) and vertebral body collapse (osteoporosis)
- Heart—Angina
- Extremities—Peripheral neuropathies and peripheral vascular disease
- Gastrointestinal (GI)—Hiatal hernia, chronic constipation, irritable bowel disease, and acute cholecystitis
- Head/neck—Temporal arteritis, cervical OA, and trigeminal neuralgia.

Pain Assessment in Older Adults

Older adults with preexisting pain pose special complications in diagnosis and management. An initial pain assessment should be performed for every new patient diagnosed with cancer, and assessments should be repeated with every new report of pain. Subsequent assessments should evaluate the effectiveness of the treatment plan; if pain is unrelieved, determine whether the pain is related to disease progression, a new cause, or cancer treatment (Jacox et al., 1994).

Initial Assessment

The initial pain assessment should include a detailed history, a physical examination with focus on the neurologic exam, a psychosocial assessment, and a diagnostic workup for pain (Jacox et al., 1994).

Subsequent Assessments

Subsequent assessments should include
- History related to pain and history of trauma
- Physical examination, including evaluation of gait, balance, and hearing
- History of pharmacologic and nonpharmacologic pain management
- Review of diagnostic data (labs, x-rays)
- Pain intensity with consideration to time of last medication dose
  - Use numerical scale or other pain intensity scale (see Figure 9.1.).
  - Use patient-generated list of pain descriptors (Stein, 1996).
  Review of systems symptom list (Patt, 1993b)
- Systemic: Anorexia, weight loss, cachexia, insomnia, and weakness
- Neurologic: Sedation, confusion, hallucinations, headache, motor weakness, altered sensation, and incontinence
- Respiratory: Dyspnea, cough, and hiccoughs
- GI: Dysphagia, nausea, vomiting, dehydration, and constipation
- Integumentary: Decubitus, dry mouth, and sore mouth
- Psychologic: Irritability, anxiety, depression, and dementia
- Genitourinary: Alteration in urinary function (Patt, 1993b)
  - Factors that exacerbate pain
  - Factors that alleviate pain
  - Meaning of pain to the patient and family
  - Cognitive screen
  - Depression screen

Figure 9.1. Pain Intensity Scales

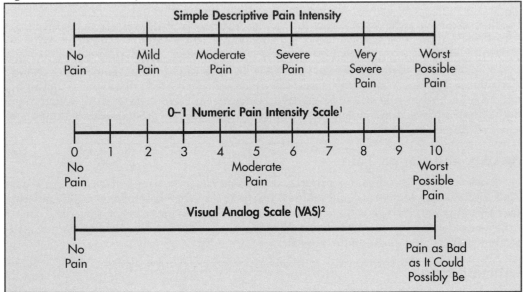

[1]If used as a graphic rating scale, a 10 cm baseline is recommended.
[2]A 10 cm baseline is recommended for VASes.
Note. From *Management of Cancer Pain. Clinical Practice Guideline #9* (p. 26), by A. Jacox, D. Carr, R. Payne et al., 1994, Rockville, MD: Agency for Human Services, Public Health Service.

- Review of activities of daily living (ADL)
- Review of instrumental ADLs (IADLs)
- List of all physicians and other healthcare professionals
- List of all medications including over-the-counter drugs (OTCs)
- IADLs, such as preparing meals, taking medications, managing finances, and using the telephone, seem to be affected by pain sooner than ADLs (Stein, 1996).

Careful assessment of recent changes in these measures is useful. Changes can be indications of complications that can impair freedom from pain (e.g., delirium, gait problems resulting in falls) (Stein, 1996).

Family

The spouse, children, and others who know the patient well should be included in the assessment process. These concerned people often will accompany the patient during the consultation. The nature of cancer and cancer pain is that it affects both patients and their significant others. Caregivers can help patients to explore concerns about pain with their healthcare providers. Patients may need knowledgeable family members to help with decision making, especially when decision-making ability is compromised by the disease (Patt, 1993b).

Depression and Cancer Pain

Major depression occurs in 20%–25% of all patients with cancer (Breitbart, Payne, & Passik, 1997). Pain and depression are a complex constellation of signs and symptoms that often co-exist in older adults with cancer. Depressed patients are more likely to have pain whether or not they are cognitively impaired (Cohen-Mansfield & Marx, 1993). Nondepressed older adults report less-intense pain (Parmalee, Katz, & Lawton, 1991). Depression increases with pain, advancing illness, and increasing functional disability (Breitbart et al.).

Depression in elderly patients with cancer is different from depression in healthy older adults. Symptoms such as anorexia, fatigue, insomnia, and weight loss are not reliable indicators of depression in patients with cancer (Breitbart et al., 1997); they may reflect disease impact rather than depression. Criteria to be substituted for the somatic criteria are tearfulness, depressive appearance, social withdrawal, decreased talkativeness, brooding, self-pity, pessimism, and lack of reactivity (Breitbart et al.). These criteria are added to the traditional depressed mood, hopelessness, worthlessness, helplessness, anhedonia, and suicidal ideation.

Anxiety and Cancer Pain

Anxiety, which is common in patients with cancer, enhances pain perception. Anxiety related to the cancer context (e.g., procedures) results in increased pain perception (Breitbart et al., 1997). Patients with cancer have reactive anxiety related to the stress of cancer and cancer therapy. Anxiety may predate the cancer diagnosis as a generalized anxiety disorder but often heightens during the illness and treatment.

Labeling Pain

Older adults are less likely to respond to the term *pain* when asked, "Do you have pain?" Patients in this population may provide more information when practitioners use other terms synonymous with pain (e.g., *discomfort, soreness, burning, aching, heaviness*) (American Geriatric Society [AGS] Panel, 1998).

Pain Assessment in Cognitively Impaired Patients With Cancer

Some cognitively impaired patients may be able to report pain at the time of assessment; however, recall often is not reliable. Cognitively impaired patients require frequent pain assessments (Stein, 1996).

Several studies of cognitively impaired elderly patients in nursing facilities have revealed high percentages of valid pain self-reports in this population (Ferrell, Ferrell, & Rivera, 1995; Parmalee, Smith, & Katz, 1993). Ferrell et al. (1995) found that 62% of residents had pain complaints; however, the patient record lacked documentation of these complaints. Tools used in assessing pain in these residents included the Present Pain Intensity Scale, the Visual Analog Scale, the Memorial Pain Card, the Rand COOP Chart, and the Verbal Scale (Ferrell et al., 1995). The researchers found that 83% of the cognitively impaired residents were able to complete at least one scale and 37% were able to complete five scales. The most successful scale was the Present Pain Intensity Scale (Melzack, 1975). Practitioners should find the pain-assessment tool that works best for each individual patient and perform pain assessment frequently to ensure adequate pain control (Stein, 1996).

Cancer Pain Management in Older Adults

The multidimensionality of the cancer pain experience requires an interdisciplinary approach to pain management. Cancer pain management is a problem of international scope, and the WHO (1990) has requested that every nation make cancer pain relief a high priority. In the United States, many organizations have worked toward this goal (Jacox et al., 1994).

Unrelieved pain causes more than just unnecessary suffering. It diminishes activity, appetite, and sleep. Pain also weakens debilitated patients and has devastating psychological effects (Jacox et al., 1994). Patients may lose hope, stop therapy, and consider or commit suicide. It devastates patients, families, and often the community.

WHO Three-Step Method

The WHO has a simple, validated, effective three-step method of pain management for cancer. It produces relief of pain in about 90% of patients with cancer.
- Step I—mild, moderate pain: Use aspirin, acetaminophen, or other nonsteroidal anti-inflammatory drugs (NSAIDs) + adjuvant therapy.
- Step II—increased pain: Add opioids, such as codeine or hydrocodone.
- Step III—persistent pain or increasing pain: Opioid is used for moderate to severe pain + nonopioid + adjuvant therapy.

If pain persists, alternative modalities such as other routes of drug administration, nerve blocks, ablative neurosurgery, and palliative radiation therapy (RT) can be tried (Jacox et al., 1994).

Pharmacologic Management of Cancer Pain in Older Adults

Pharmacologic management is the mainstay of therapy for cancer pain. Avoidance of side effects is an ever-present concern in pain management in older adults; however, overconcern may lead to undertreatment and unnecessary suffering.

Great variation exists in the effects of pain medications in older adults. In general, starting doses of morphine should be lower in the older population, and dose intervals may need to be longer. Figure 9.2 provides additional prescribing guidelines.

NSAIDs

NSAIDs are useful in the treatment of arthritis pain, which is common in older adults. NSAIDs may alleviate inflammatory pain and musculoskeletal pain and may be used to potentiate the effects of opiates (Kelly & Payne, 1993). NSAIDs are useful in the treatment of pain caused by bone metastases because NSAIDs inhibit prostaglandin release, which can cause pain. A risk of bleeding is present with the use of NSAIDs, especially in elderly patients. Approximately 90% of NSAID-induced fatal hemorrhages occur in the stomach and in patients older than age 60 (Kelly & Payne). NSAIDs can cause renal and GI toxicities because of impaired metabolism and excretion (Kelly & Payne). The new COX-2 inhibitors appear useful in elderly patients. Patients may take misoprostol (Cytotec®, G.D. Searle & Co., Chicago, IL) or an H2 inhibitor to decrease gastric effects (Stein, 1997), and GI irritation also may be minimized if patients take NSAIDs with food or milk. Other possible side effects include sodium and water retention, confusion, agitation, headache, hallucinations, and decreased effect of some antihypertensives. See Table 9.1 for dosing information associated with specific NSAIDs.

It is not unusual for one NSAID to be ineffective in treating pain in the elderly patient with cancer. A positive response may be achieved by switching to another NSAID before changing to another classification of drugs. Patients should be monitored for toxic effects of NSAIDs for at least three months after treatment is discontinued, as a GI bleed could occur at any time. Baseline hemoglobin, hematocrit, BUN, creatinine, and stool specimen guaiac levels should be obtained every three months.

Aspirin is useful as a treatment for mild to moderate pain and has good anti-inflammatory effects. It is not advisable for use in frail elderly patients because it causes bleeding. GI bleed

Figure 9.2. Guidelines for Prescribing Analgesics in Elderly Patients With Cancer

- Medical history should include concurrent medications, prior adverse reactions, and concomitant illnesses.
- Resist prescribing without a diagnosis.
- Start low and increase slowly.
- Continually review prescription medications and over-the-counter drugs.
- Decrease or remove medications when indicated.
- Evaluate compliance continuously.
- Patients may decrease the dose or omit drugs; the drug may be prescribed in a hospital setting at the usual dose, resulting in toxic levels.
- Avoid intramuscular injections in elderly patients; rectal administration of drugs is an acceptable alternative, especially morphine.
- Essential concepts of the WHO Drug Approach for Cancer:
  - By mouth rather than parenteral
  - By the clock, not as needed or requested
  - By the WHO Ladder
  - Individualized to each patient
  - Attention to detail

Note. Based on information from Fulmer, Mion, & Bottrell, 1996; Gloth, 1996; WHO, 1996.

is common. Side effects from high doses of aspirin include tinnitus, dizziness, confusion, drowsiness, and nausea and vomiting. GI bleeding and anemia also can occur from the direct action of aspirin on the mucosa of the stomach.

Acetaminophen is equivalent to aspirin as an analgesic and antipyretic but has little anti-inflammatory effect. Acetaminophen is safe to use in older adults. The highest recommended daily dose is 4,000 mg; however, this dose should be lower in frail elderly patients (Gloth, 1996). Liver and renal damage can occur with long-term use and high doses. Liver toxicity is increased in people who also use alcohol. Acetaminophen is found in many preparations. Patients should be instructed to read the ingredients in OTCs to avoid increasing the total dose of acetaminophen.

Bromfenac sodium is a newer NSAID that is indicated for pain management. It is an analgesic, antipyretic, and anti-inflammatory agent but is recommended for short-term use (i.e., fewer than 10 days).

COX-2 inhibitors are a new class of drugs that are thought to relieve pain as well as aspirin and other NSAIDs while producing no side effects (Gorman, 1998). The drugs block COX-2, which triggers pain and inflammation. Unlike aspirin and other NSAIDs, the new drugs do not block COX-1, which is a protector of stomach lining and platelet regulation.

Opiates for Treatment of Cancer in Older Adults

For Step II of the WHO cancer pain management guideline, codeine, given by mouth, is an acceptable first drug for use in the treatment of moderate pain in older adults. However, its usefulness is limited by its constipating side effect, which is more pronounced than with other narcotic agents. Codeine is especially effective for mild to moderate pain and is used in combination with acetaminophen or aspirin. Codeine has an antitussive effect, which may be useful to relieve cough associated with some tumors. The usual dose of codeine is 15–60 mg q 4–6 h. A dose of 200 mg of codeine is equal to 30 mg of morphine (Stein, 1997). Codeine can be administered with milk to reduce GI distress.

Table 9.1. Nonsteroidal Anti-Inflammatory Drugs (NSAIDs) for Older Adults With Cancer

Drug	Starting Dose	Maximum Dose	Comments
Acetaminophen	325 mg bid	4,000 mg/24h	Antipyretic, negative anti-inflammatory
Aspirin	325 mg bid	4,000 mg/24h	Platelet effects irreversible
Ibuprofen	200 mg q 6–8 h	800 mg/8h	—
Naproxen	250 mg q 12 h	500 mg/12h	Start NSAIDs low dose and around-the-clock.
Ketoprofen	75 mg tid/50 mg qid	300 mg/24h	Short half-life
Choline magnesium trisalicylate	1,000 mg–1,500 mg bid	5,500 mg/24h	Does not affect platelet aggregation

Note. Based on information from American Geriatrics Society Panel, 1998.

Morphine and other strong opioids, such as oxycodone and fentanyl, are the drugs of choice for the treatment of severe pain in older adults with cancer. There is no ceiling to the analgesic effect of morphine. Its half-life is two hours, and the duration of analgesia is approximately four hours. Slow-release forms have been shown to be safe and effective and are administered only two or three times per day. Patients taking the slow-release morphine appear to have fewer problems with nausea and vomiting as a side effect (Vanegas, 1998). However, oral morphine is not as effective as other delivery methods (Vanegas). Patients with known renal disease must be monitored for side effects because of poor excretion, which results in an increased accumulation of morphine (Kelly & Payne, 1993). Figure 9.3 lists medications to avoid in older patients.

Psychological addiction to opiates is very uncommon in older adults. However, physical dependency occurs with long-term use; therefore, weaning must be done slowly to prevent withdrawal symptoms.

Major side effects of opiates include respiratory depression, constipation, and urine retention. Patients may be more prone to falls because of sedation and confusion caused by opiate use. Less-common side effects include sweating, pruritus, hallucinations, hyperalgesia, myoclonus, and "cognitive failure" (Vanegas, 1998). Patients should be monitored closely for side effects during titration. Nursing interventions for patients who are taking opiates for analgesia include the following.

- Assess respiration and mental status.
- Prevent constipation by starting a bowel regimen of laxatives, stool softeners, increased dietary fiber, and water.
- Monitor intake and output.
- Assess skin.
- Assess gait and balance.
- Monitor for sedation and confusion.
- Evaluate home environment for safety.

Transdermal Administration of Analgesia

Fentanyl is a very potent synthetic narcotic that typically is administered transdermally (Gever, 1998). It is useful in patients who are unable to take oral medications and those who have chronic rather than acute pain. The transdermal patch can be placed on the thigh, abdo-

Figure 9.3. Medications to Avoid in Older Adults

- **Meperidine:** Its metabolite has a prolonged half-life, which accumulates, is toxic, and can result in agitation and seizures not reversed with naloxone (Kelly & Payne, 1993).
- **Pentazocine:** This drug is known to cause hallucinations in older adults, and it has agonist-antagonist properties (Gloth, 1996).
- **Levorphanol:** This drug has a prolonged elimination half-life beyond the analgesic effect. It may have increased sedation and respiratory depressant effects (Gloth).
- **Methadone:** This drug also has a prolonged half-life beyond its analgesic effect (Gloth).
- **Cimetidine:** This drug can cause confusion.
- **Promethazine hydrochloride given with narcotics:** This combination appears to be antianalgesic; for nausea, give hydroxyzine hydrochloride or hydroxyzine pamoate, which seem to have analgesic effects (Stein, 1997b).

men, chest, or upper arm (Gever). The site should be rotated when a new patch is applied because skin reactions have been reported in about 4% of patients (Manfredi, Weinstein, Chandler, & Payne, 1997). Fentanyl is delivered through the skin over 72 hours, but the effects may last longer in older adults (AGS Panel, 1998). It may take 18–24 hours to reach a peak effect after the patch is initially applied, and it may take up to six days to obtain a steady state of analgesia when the dose is increased. Fentanyl patches are available in four strengths: 25, 50, 75, and 100 mcg/hour. A 25 mcg patch is roughly equivalent to 30 mg of long-acting morphine administered twice a day (Baumann, 1997).

Patients who experience breakthrough pain (end-of-dose failure) or incident pain while using fentanyl patches should have an immediate-release oral morphine available. If more than four breakthrough medication doses are needed, the dose of the patch should be increased.

Intraspinal Opioids

For patients whose side effects have not been managed by conventional means, intraspinal opioids are a choice for reversible analgesia for somatic or visceral pain with a favorable risk-to-benefit ratio in terminally ill patients with cancer (Waldman, Leak, Kennedy, & Patt, 1993). Epidural (peridural) and intrathecal (subarachnoid) are the two routes used. The advantage of intraspinal opioids is that they do not affect selectivity, motor, sensory, and sympathetic systems (Waldman et al.). Postoperatively, epidural opioids have demonstrated fewer postoperative pulmonary complications than systemic narcotics (Ballantyne et al., 1998). Dull, constant pain (slow, second pain of C-fibers) is most amenable to intraspinal opioid therapy, while patients with acute, sharp, breakthrough pain (first pain) find less relief (Waldman et al.).

Potential side effects of opiates such as morphine, hydromorphone, and fentanyl administered directly into the central nervous system (CNS) are respiratory depression, nausea and vomiting, urinary retention, pruritus, and marked sedation (Baumann, 1997). Intrathecal administration produces analgesia at lower doses and with fewer side effects (Baumann).

Patient-Controlled Analgesia

Patient-controlled analgesia (PCA) provides older patients with cancer and caregivers some control over pain management (Waldman et al., 1993). Some patients and caregivers may be overwhelmed with the technology and increase in responsibility and require additional time and education about PCA before becoming comfortable with this administration technique. Even with instruction, some patients and caregivers may surrender control and not accept the responsibility.

According to Waldman et al. (1993), PCA can
- Eliminate the need for breakthrough doses.
- Decrease anxiety in patients with breakthrough pain.
- Decrease the overall dose needed.
- Increase the patient's sense of control.

General guidelines for PCA opiate use in older adults include the following (Kelly & Payne, 1993).
- Use opiates with a short half-life, such as morphine and hydromorphone.
- Avoid using methadone, levorphanol, meperidine, and propoxyphene.
- Administer medication around the clock (ATC).
- If pain persists at the end of the specified time period, shorten the dose interval rather than increasing the drug dose.
- Anticipate side effects, especially constipation, sedation, and confusion.
- Use adjuvant medications (e.g., NSAIDs, antiemetics, hydroxyzine).

- Begin PCA with a lower dose, and titrate up as needed.
- Use equianalgesic information when changing medications or the route of delivery (Kingdon, Stanley, & Kizior, 1998). For example, 3 mg of morphine given epidurally is the equivalent of 30 mg given orally or 10 mg given parenterally. A dose of 1 mg hydromorphone administered epidurally is equivalent to 7.5 mg given orally or 1.5 mg given parenterally (Skobel, 1996) (see Table 9.2).
- Use adjuvant medications for primary pain control in neuropathies or bone pain, to treat opioid side effects, and to alleviate psychological distress (Stein, 1997).

Tricyclic Antidepressants

Tricyclic antidepressants (TCAs) are found to be useful in the treatment of neuropathic pain. Their analgesic effect may be related to decreasing depression and mood improvement

Table 9.2. Dose Equivalents for Opioid Analgesics in Opioid-Naïve Adults Weighing Less Than 50 kg

Drug	Equianalgesic Dose		Usual Starting Dose for Moderate/Severe Pain	
	Oral	Parenteral	Oral	Parenteral
Morphine	30 mg q 3–4 h around-the-clock	10 mg q 3–4 h	0.3 mg/kg q 3–4 h	0.1 mg/kg q 3–4 h
	60 mg q 3–4 h single dose or intermittent dosing	N/A	N/A	N/A
Morphine, controlled-release	90–120 mg q 12 h	N/A	N/A	N/A
Hydromorphone	7.5 mg q 3–4 h	1.5 mg q 3–4 h	0.06 mg/kg q 3–4 h	0.015 mg/ kg q 3–4 h
Levorphanol	4 mg q 6–8 h	2 mg q 6–8 h	0.04 mg/kg q 6–8 h	0.02 mg/ kg q 6–8 h
Codeine (with asprin or acetaminophen)	180–200 mg q 3–4 h	130 mg q 3–4 h	0.5–1 mg/kg q 3–4 h	N/A
Hydrocodone	30 mg q 3–4h	N/A	0.2 mg/kg q 3–4 h	N/A
Oxycodone	30 mg q 3–4 h	N/A	0.2 mg/kg q 3–4 h	N/A

Note. Based on information from Jacox et al., 1994

(Kelly & Payne). TCAs are not effective in treatment of musculoskeletal pain. Higher doses of the medication are needed for treatment of depression superimposed on cancer pain, while doses lower than those used for depression can be used to treat pain, especially neuropathic pain. Norpramin appears to be better tolerated by older adults and has fewer anticholinergic effects than some of the other TCAs (Kelly & Payne).

Anticholinergic side effects of TCAs can include constipation, blurred vision, dry mouth, urinary retention, and sedation. Patients with glaucoma and benign prostatic hypertrophy should be monitored closely if TCAs are used. TCAs can cause arrhythmias, cognitive changes, and orthostatic hypotension, resulting in falls (Gloth, 1996). Patients who are taking TCAs should be monitored with electrocardiogram and blood pressure evaluations. TCAs should be administered at night, and doses should be increased slowly over three to four weeks. The medication should be continued for at least four to six weeks before discontinuing therapy because of a failure to respond (Kelly & Payne, 1993). Table 9.3 provides additional dosage guidelines.

Analgesic Anticonvulsants and Other Adjuvant Medications

Anticonvulsants are useful in relieving paroxysms of lancinating pain (Manfredi et al., 1997). They can be used with stimulants and antihistamines for additional analgesic effects. Table 9.4 lists specific anticonvulsants used for pain management.

Stein (1997b) suggested a number of other adjuvant agents that may be useful in pain management. Phenothiazines also may have analgesic effects in addition to use for the treatment of nausea and vomiting (Stein, 1997). Haloperidol, chlorpromazine, and prochlorpemazine are suggested for use with older adults. Chlorpromazine also is useful for the treatment of hiccoughs and coughs. Anxiolytics and short-acting benzodiazepines are useful, as well. Table 9.5 lists additional adjuvant medications.

EMLA® Cream (AstraZeneca, Wilmington, DE) has been found to be useful as a topical anesthetic for painful procedures (Hines, 1995). The cream is applied, using gloves, two hours before breast needle localizations, implanted port injections, and IV sticks. The maximum anesthetic effect is four hours. Use is contraindicated in patients who are sensitive to lidocaine (Hines).

Undertreatment

Older adults with cancer are at risk for undertreatment of pain. In one study of more than 1,300 patients with cancer, age 70 years or older was shown to be a predictor of inadequate pain management (Cleeland, Gonin, & Hatfield, 1994). Elderly patients with cancer may not receive good pain management until their pain becomes very severe or their disease is very advanced. The National Hospice Study examined hospice care and conventional cancer care and found that hospice care provided better pain and symptom control and showed higher patient satisfaction (Mor, Greer, & Kastenbaum, 1988). The nonhospice patients did not receive adequate

Table 9.3. Tricyclic Antidepressants for Pain Relief in Older Adults

Drug	Starting Dose	Usual Daily Dose	Comments
Amitriptyline	10 mg	75–100 mg	Sedating
Imipramine	10 mg	50–200 mg	Anticholinergic
Doxapine	10 mg	75–150 mg	—
Nortriptyline	10–25 mg	75–100 mg	—
Desipramine	10–25 mg	75–200 mg	Fewer side effects

Table 9.4. Anticonvulsants Used for Pain Management

Drug	Starting Dose	Maintenance Dose	Comments
Carbamazepine	100–200 mg qd, give 100 bid	300–800 mg qd	Sedation, nausea, ataxia, congestive heart failure, liver toxicity, and arrhythmia
Phenytoin	100 mg	150–600 mg in 2–3 divided doses	Similar side effects and less effective
Valproic acid	15 mg/kg/day in 3–4 divided doses	60 mg/kg/day in divided doses	Nausea and vomiting, tremor, hepatotoxicity, decreased platelets, and less sedating
Clonazepam	0.5–1 mg	10–20 mg	Sedation and ataxia

Note. Based on information from Kelly & Payne, 1993.

pain management as compared to the ATC management of hospice patients. Further, the Agency for Health Care Policy and Research's cancer pain management guidelines (Jacox et al., 1994) indicate that older adults are an "at-risk" group because of inadequate nursing education regarding the management of pain in this population.

Family Factors

Cancer pain management is influenced by family factors (Ferrell, Ferrell, Rhiner, & Grant, 1991). Caregivers tend to estimate pain in their loved ones at higher levels than patients do. In one study, using a scale of 0–100, patients' estimates of pain averaged 45.5, while caregivers' estimates averaged 69.9. Caregivers estimated their own distress from patients' pain at 77.4 (Ferrell et al.).

Surgery, Radiation, and Chemotherapy for Pain Management

Although 70% of patients should attain management of pain via pharmacologic control, 30% will require alternate therapies (Patt & Jain, 1993). The primary control for cancer-related pain is treatment directed toward control of the disease itself using surgery, RT, or chemotherapy or control of a disease-related event, such as using antibiotics for infection, anti-inflammatory agents to reduce inflammation, or antihyperuricemic agents to control the symptoms of gout (Kurman, 1993).

Invasive Treatments to Manage Cancer Pain

Local Pain Blocks

Acute herpes zoster is common in elderly patients with cancer, and early resolution can prevent post-herpetic neuralgia (PHN) (Raj, 1993). In addition to pharmacologic therapy, nerve blocks with local infiltration may be beneficial in relieving PHN. While clinicians report nearly

Table 9.5. Adjuvant Medications

Drug	Recommended Dose	Comments
Antihistamines Hydroxyzine	25–50 mg po	Analgesic, antiemetic, and mild sedative; not used in patients with glaucoma
Benzodiazepines Alprazolam Lorazepam	 0.125–0.5 mg tid 0.5–1.0 mg tid	No analgesia; may potentiate opioids
Stimulants Caffeine	100–300 mg qd	Enhances analgesia; decreases sedative effect of opioids
Steroids Dexamethasone	16 mg qd x 2–3 days; 4 mg qd maintenance	Decreases edema; enhances analgesia

100% success in reducing PHN in younger patients with cancer with subcutaneous injections of 0.2% triamcinolone in normal saline into painful sites of eruption, a high percentage of older adults continue the course of PHN (Raj).

Neural Blocks

Neural blocks are used to manage intractable pain. They are most applicable for pain that is well characterized, localized, or visceral but are not useful for vague pain syndromes characterized by multifocal aches and pains (Patt & Jain, 1993). Referral to a pain clinic or anesthesiologist for evaluation is appropriate. Neural blocks usually are given to patients with a short (i.e., less than 60 months) life expectancy because the analgesic effects subside, leaving the patient with a painful numbness.

Orthopedic Management

Painful long-bone pathological fractures from bone metastases may be treated surgically. The pain can be reduced and the bone stabilized with a metal plate or rod. The surgical intervention is followed by RT (Rosier, 1993). There is an increased rate of success with pain reduction and return to function with this treatment plan. Pathological fractures near a hip, knee, or shoulder can be corrected with a joint replacement using a prosthesis. Bone grafts usually are performed in patients with cancers associated with long survival rates, such as breast and prostate cancers (Rosier).

Palliative Chemotherapy

Dramatic tumor response and alleviation of tumor associated pain are observed even in patients with advanced disease (Kurman, 1993). Criteria for determination of candidacy for palliative chemotherapy include the following.

- Toxicity of therapy and the patient's ability to tolerate toxicity—The performance status of the patient, not the patient's age, should be used to determine the patient's candidacy for this treatment. Reliable performance status measures include the Eastern Cooperative Oncology Group (ECOG) scale (Zubrod, Schneiderman, & Frei, 1960) and the Karnofsky Scale (Karnofsky, Abelman, & Craver, 1948).
- Tumor histology—All systemic chemotherapies have side effects, so therapy may have an adverse effect on the patient's quality of life. Chemotherapy only should be used if there is a possibility of positive treatment results. For example, chemotherapy for non-small cell lung cancer has marginal efficacy and significant toxicity; therefore, it may not be an appropriate treatment for this patient population.
- Patient history of prior therapy—Tumors develop resistance to the effects of drugs after multiple courses of chemotherapy. Bone marrow depletion may result earlier in the course of treatment if the patient has been exposed to the chemotherapy agent in the past.

Palliative Radiation

RT is the mainstay of pain control in patients with bone metastases (Rosier, 1993). RT is highly effective for bone metastases associated with lung, breast, and prostate cancers. Treatment usually is administered in high doses over a short time period (Ashby, 1993). Radioisotopes also may be used for pain relief, but the onset of relief is delayed (Ashby).

RT may be useful for relief of pain originating from the nerve root and soft-tissue infiltration. RT also may be a useful therapeutic tool for pain associated with apical lung cancer and brachial plexus invasion and the severe pain of pelvic recurrence from inoperable rectal adenocarcinoma (Ashby, 1993).

The radiation effect in older adults is increased 10%–15% in normal tissues (Cohen, 1994). They tend to experience an increased incidence of nausea and vomiting when compared to younger adults receiving RT (Cohen).

Noninvasive Pain Management in Older Adults

Older adults with chronic cancer pain may prefer nonpharmacologic methods of pain control. Heat and vibration are especially useful in this patient population (Lueckenotte, 1996). These techniques may be used alone or in combination with pharmacologic therapy. Noninvasive, nonpharmacologic treatment may be categorized as cognitive/behavioral and physical. Cognitive/behavioral therapy means changing the perception of pain, altering pain behaviors, and increasing the patient's sense of control over the pain. Physical treatments are to increase comfort, improve function, alter the physical response, and decrease the fear associated with pain-related immobility (Jacox et al., 1994).

Cognitive/Behavioral Therapies

Cognitive/behavioral therapies may be used for acute or chronic pain. Positive self-statements (self-talk) help patients to cope with present pain. Patients are encouraged to think that "tomorrow will be better" and "soon this will be over." Self-talk is useful, especially for short-lived, acute pains such as the pain associated with a procedure. Teaching patients about the procedure and the length of time that they can expect to experience pain may be helpful when the information is given prior to the procedure.

- Autogenic training uses mental phrases to decrease sympathetic activity. Patients assume a relaxed position and concentrate on feelings of warmth, heaviness, or a slowed heart rate and respiration. Mentally, patients say, "My legs are heavy and warm" or "My breathing is slow and calm" (Millard, 1993).
- Meditation is the development of a calm, receptive mental state achieved by resting in a quiet environment and focusing on an object or word. Patients breathe slowly, adopt a passive attitude, and exhale while focusing on a word such as *calm* (Millard, 1993).
- Imagery can be used alone or with autogenic training. Patients create a vivid mental picture, such as a setting sun, a beach with blowing winds and sand, or any setting that evokes pleasure and peaceful feelings (Millard, 1993).
- Relaxation is used to alter physiologic activity (Millard, 1993). Relaxation treatments such as distraction also help to decrease anxiety. Relaxation and guided imagery can be used together to enhance the results.
- Progressive relaxation is alternating contraction and relaxation of muscle groups. This is useful in procedures related to cancer symptom control. Patients can be taught a sequential head-to-toe or hand-to-shoulder relaxation strategy (Millard, 1993).
- Jaw relaxation and abdominal breathing often are used to manage tension. Patients should repeat breathing cycles 8–10 times. The jaw is dropped, and patients are instructed to perform deep, rhythmic inhalations followed by slow exhalation.
- Distraction strategies include watching TV, listening to the radio, visiting with family and friends, and reading. These techniques may be useful for relief of mild pain. Distraction is used to change the attention focus by occupying the mind with something other than the pain. Distraction strategies must be individualized to each patient. Other distractions that can be used include visual stimuli; auditory or tactile distractions, such as pet therapy; and involvement in projects, such as games, puzzles, and journals (Millard, 1993).
- Cognitive therapy is a strategy used to modify patients' appraisals of pain when it is "threatening" (Millard, 1993). It counters depressive thinking and may reduce suffering. The process begins with educating patients about pain and the role of cognition in pain perception. Patients track and record episodes of pain and distress and then interpret the thoughts that accompany the episodes with their nurses. Relaxation methods are incorporated to divert patients' attention from the pain. Eventually, patients develop a sense of mastery over the pain.
- Hypnosis has been used in the management of pain associated with breast cancer (Classen, Hermanson, & Spiegel, 1994). It shares features of deep concentration, imagery, and breathing exercises with other behavior modification therapies (Millard, 1993). Unlike the other therapies discussed, however, hypnosis usually requires professional assistance. Self-hypnosis begins with relaxation, closing the eyes, focusing on the pain, and seeing its color, shape, and size. Patients then "project" the pain into space and make it bigger, make it smaller, and then let it be any size. They change the color of pain and then put it back. When complete, patients can open their eyes (Millard).
- Biofeedback is a behavioral intervention, the purpose of which is to train patients to modify involuntary physiologic activities, such as respiration and muscle activity (spasm). Little evidence of success with the use of this strategy in patients with cancer is available. Biofeedback requires considerable motivation to be effective.
- Group therapy/family therapy can be used successfully to help patients with cancer to deal with the pain, depression, and anxiety that can accompany cancer (Millard, 1993). Weekly group therapy combined with self-hypnosis has been shown to be beneficial for pain relief (Millard). This approach increases one's sense of control over the threat of cancer and the pain.

- Education of both patients and families can be helpful. Patients and family members may fear the use of opiate analgesia and the tolerance, addiction, and respiratory depression that can accompany it. Families also may fear that opiates will hasten death (Ferrell, 1998).
- Music therapy is another method used to reduce pain (Bral, 1998). It is a distraction technique that promotes relaxation and decreases anxiety. Selections of music are based upon patient preferences. Music affects mood and may stimulate endorphins to modulate pain transmission and decrease pain perception.

Physical Therapies

Various forms of physical therapy can be used for pain management. These strategies include cutaneous stimulation with heat and cold, massage, exercise, acupuncture, and counterstimulation such as transcutaneous electrical nerve stimulation (TENS).
- Heat is known to decrease pain and discomfort by increasing blood flow to the skin and superficial tissues, increasing oxygen and nutrient delivery, and decreasing joint stiffness by increasing the elasticity of muscles (Jacox et al., 1994). Some of the delivery modalities include hot water bottles, heating pads, compresses, tub baths, soaks, and heat lamps. Cold reduces pain and inflammation and edema after an acute injury. It may reduce muscle spasm not alleviated by heat treatments (Jacox et al.) and alter the pain threshold (Millard, 1993). Cold decreases transmission of pain stimuli and decreases the release of bradykinins, histamines, and serotonin. Delivery modalities include ice bags, cold packs, compresses, cool soaks, and cool baths. People often have an individual preference for heat *or* cold for pain relief.
- Massage is a patterned motion of light to deep pressure (as in rubbing, kneading, stroking, or smoothing) used to promote relaxation and decrease anxiety. Massage stimulates A fibers competing at the gates for transmission and closes the gates to painful stimuli. All forms of touch usually are pleasurable to older adults (Ebersole & Hess, 1998); however, individuals may have specific preferences of creams and salves used in massage. Massage should be used carefully in patients with bone metastases, as they are at high risk for fractures.
- Exercise or physical therapy can help to maintain or improve function, prevent stiffness, relieve muscle spasms, and generally increase one's sense of well-being. Most elderly patients with cancer should be referred for consultation with a physical therapist. Physical therapy usually is not used for the management of acute pain or moderate chronic pain without premedication.
- Acupressure is manual pressure applied to acupuncture sites. Acupuncture is insertion of needles at acupuncture sites; the needles are then manually twirled or electrically stimulated. The stimulation competes for placement on pain receptor sites closing the gates to pain (Millard, 1993). Acupressure and acupuncture should be performed by a professional certified in these treatments.
- TENS is a safe, noninvasive, relatively inexpensive modality that can be used in conjunction with other therapies. It has been found to be useful in pain control in older adults (Eiman, Anderson, Donela, & Silverman, 1996). It is has been used effectively for neuropathic pain, spinal pain, and neuralgias. A two-to-four-week trial will determine if the treatment is effective.

Other Therapies

Therapeutic and healing touch, herbal remedies, and humor may be of benefit in managing pain in older patients. These therapies can be used in conjunction with all other therapies.
- Therapeutic touch is a therapy developed by nurses that may be used in any setting (Millard, 1993). The therapy directs energy to the patient to give pain relief and promote healing. No physical contact occurs between the therapist and patient. The therapist "centers," reaching

a meditative state that is sensitive to the patient's needs, and assesses the patient's energy flow with hand scans bilaterally to detect differences in temperature, energy, and rhythm. Therapeutic touch is said to restore the balance of energy using vivid visualization (Millard).

- Herbal remedies are thought by some to have beneficial effects. St. John's wort is believed to have an antidepressant effect, as are gotu kola, ginseng, skullcap, and lavender (Eliopoulos, 1997).
- Humor often is used as a distraction from pain. However, it is less likely to be a coping mechanism used by older adults facing threats and losses from cancer and pain (McCrae, 1984).

Barriers to Pain Management

Older adults are at risk for undertreatment of pain. Most research on pain and cancer pain is conducted on younger patients, and the results are generalized to elderly patients. In fact, few older adults, especially the oldest old, are treated in pain clinics, which report much of the information available on pain. This is interesting when one considers that older adults have an increased incidence of chronic pain (Corran, Gibson, Farrell, & Helm, 1994).

Age

Age is a predictor of inadequate pain management. Cleeland et al. (1994) reported a study of more than 1,300 outpatients with metastatic cancer and found that age 70 and older was a predictor of inadequate pain management.

Reporting

A major barrier to cancer pain management is the older patient's reluctance to report pain problems. Reasons given may include the following.
- The complaint might distract the doctor from treating the cancer.
- The patient may fear that the cancer is getting worse.
- The patient may want to be seen by the healthcare provider as a "good patient," not a complaining patient (Miaskowski, 1997).
- Pain is considered to be part of aging (Ebersole & Hess, 1998).
- Healthcare professionals may incorrectly assume that elderly patients will spontaneously report their pain (Ebersole & Hess, 1998).

Education

Many barriers to good pain management exist. Educational barriers are among the most important—yet they can be remedied (Stein & Ferrell, 1996). Most nurses are not well educated in the care of elderly patients. In the face of the changing demographics of the population, gerontology is not yet treated as a nursing specialty in schools of nursing, as are pediatrics and obstetrics (Luggen, 1997). Oncology patient care is integrated in the nursing curricula, but nurses may never have a continuing education program to update this knowledge. Education levels of patients and family members also may cause difficulty in managing the patients' pain, especially in patients who are receiving home care.

Myths

A number of myths about pain in older adults interfere with good pain management. One myth is that older adults who are treated for pain may become addicted. An important legal case of inadequate pain management related to pain myths in a nursing home ended with a $15 million verdict against the nursing home for failing to provide adequate pain relief to a patient (Ferrell et al., 1990). In this case, the patient was a 75-year-old man with stage III metastatic prostate cancer with pathological fractures who recently had been discharged from a hospital with a terminal diagnosis. He was prescribed morphine, with the goal of pain relief. The nurse caregiver decided that the patient was addicted to the morphine and substituted a mild tranquilizer and withheld or delayed the prescribed morphine. The courts ruled in favor of the patient.

Race

Ebersole and Hess (1998) reported some culture-specific responses to pain that may inhibit good pain management. These include patients minimizing pain reports to significant others; using pain to elicit sympathy; controlling the expression of pain; appearing calm and unemotional; crying and moaning when in pain; withdrawing when in severe pain; seeking attention; avoiding pain-relief measures, believing that they indicate weakness; wanting and expecting quick pain relief; and accepting pain for long periods of time before requesting help (Ebersole & Hess).

Gender

Nurses believe that gender differences affect sensitivity to pain and have thought that women should receive smaller doses of narcotic analgesics than men (Ebersole & Hess, 1998). Recent information suggests that gender-related pain perception does occur and that it is physiologic (Vallerand, 1995). Women appear to be more sensitive to pain.

Finances

Financial problems or below-poverty-level incomes inhibit patients' ability to purchase desired medications for pain management. Patients may end up choosing between such necessities as food and rent and pain medications (Stein, 1997).

Conclusion

Nurses need to assist patients in developing active coping strategies. These may include planning distractions, such as TV watching, or seeking help with hypnosis. Passive coping is related to general psychological distress and depression. Education is one of the most important tools nurses can use to assist patients and families to control pain and reduce suffering. A structured pain-education program can decrease pain intensity, decrease perception of pain, increase the use of pain medications, reduce anxiety and fear of addiction, and improve sleep (Ferrell, Rhiner, & Ferrell, 1993). Development of a pain-education program is within the scope of nursing practice.

References

American Geriatrics Society Panel. (1998). The management of chronic pain in older persons. *Journal of the American Geriatric Society, 46,* 635–651.

Ashby, M. (1993). Radiotherapy in palliation of cancer. In R.B. Patt (Ed.), *Cancer pain* (pp. 235–249). Philadelphia: Lippincott.

Ballantyne, J.C., Carr, D.B., deFerranti, S., Suarez, T., Lauo, J., Chalmers, T.C., Angelillo, I.F., & Mosteller, F. (1998). The comparative effects of postoperative analgesic therapies on pulmonary outcome: Cumulative meta-analyses of randomized controlled trials. *Anesthesia & Analgesia, 86*, 598–612.

Baumann, T.J. (1997). Pain management. In J.T. Dipiro (Ed.), *Pharmacotherapy: A pathophysiologic approach* (3rd ed.) (pp. 1259–1278). Stamford, CT: Appleton & Lange.

Bernabei, R., Gambassi, G., Lapane, K., Landi, F., Gatsonis, C., & Dunlop, R. (1998). Management of pain in elderly patients with cancer. *JAMA, 279*, 1877–1882.

Bowsher, D., Rigge, M., & Sopp, L. (1991). Prevalence of chronic pain in the British population: A telephone survey of 1037 households. *Pain Clinics, 4*, 223–230.

Bral, E. (1998). Caring for adults with chronic cancer pain. *American Journal of Nursing, 98*(4), 24–28.

Brattberg, G., Parker, M., & Thorslund, M. (1996). The prevalence of pain among the oldest old in Sweden. *Pain, 67*, 29–34.

Breitbart, W., Payne, D., & Passik, S. (1997). Psychiatric and psychological aspects of cancer pain. In W.C.V. Parris (Ed.), *Cancer pain management* (pp. 253–277). Boston: Butterworth-Heinemann.

Chakour, M.C., Gibson, S.J., Bradbeer, M., & Helme, R.D. (1996). The effect of age on A delta and C-fibre thermal pain perception. *Pain, 64*, 143–152.

Classen, C., Hermanson, K., & Spiegel, C. (1994). Psychotherapy, stress and survival in breast cancer. In C. Lewis, C.O. Sullivan, & J. Barraclough (Eds.), *The psychoimmunology of cancer* (pp. 124–156). New York: Oxford Medical Publishers.

Cleeland, C.S., Gonin, R., & Hatfield, A. (1994). Pain and its treatment in outpatients with metastatic cancer. *New England Journal of Medicine, 330*, 592–596.

Cohen, H. (1994). Oncology and aging: General principles of cancer treatment in the elderly. In W. Hazzard, E. Berman, J. Blass, W. Ettinger, & J. Holter (Eds.), *Principles of geriatric medicine and gerontology* (pp. 77–94). St. Louis: McGraw-Hill.

Cohen-Mansfield, J., & Marx, M.S. (1993). Pain and depression in the nursing home. *Journal of Gerontology, 48*, 96–97.

Corran, T., Gibson, S., Farrell, M., & Helm, R. (1994). Comparison of chronic pain experiences between young and elderly patients. In G. Gebhart, D. Hammond, & T. Jenson (Eds.), *Proceedings of the 7th World Congress on Pain* (Vol. 2) (pp. 895–906). Seattle: IASP Press.

Crook, J., Rideout, E., & Browne, G. (1984). The prevalence of pain complaints in a general population. *Pain, 18*, 299–314.

Ebersole, P., & Hess, P. (1998). *Toward healthy aging* (5th ed.). St. Louis: Mosby.

Elman, M., Anderson, S., Donela, H., & Silverman, M. (1996). Geriatric pain management. In E. Salerno & J. Willens (Eds.), *Pain management handbook* (pp. 375–404). St. Louis: Mosby.

Eliopoulos, C. (1997). *Gerontological nursing* (4th ed.). Philadelphia: Lippincott.

Ferrell, B.R. (1998). End-of-life care. How well do we serve our patients? *Nursing 98, 28*(9), 58–60.

Ferrell, B., Rhiner, R., & Ferrell, B.A. (1993). Development and implementation of a patient education program. *Cancer, 72*, 3426–3432.

Ferrell, B.A., Ferrell, B.R., Rhiner, M., & Grant, M. (1991, September). *Family factors influence cancer pain management.* Paper presented at the First Asian-Pacific Symposium on Pain Control, Sydney, Australia.

Ferrell, B.A., Ferrell, B.R., & Rivera, L. (1995). Cognitively impaired nursing home patients. *Journal of Symptom Management, 10*, 591–595.

Ferrell, B.A., Ferrell, B.R, & Osterweil, D. (1990). Pain in the nursing home. *Journal of the American Geriatrics Society, 38*, 409–414.

Foley, K.M. (1985). Treatment of cancer pain. *New England Journal of Medicine, 313*, 84–95.

Fulmer, T., Mion, L., & Bottrell, M. (1996). Pain management protocol. NICHE Faculty. *Geriatric Nursing, 17*, 222–227.

Gever, M.P. (1998). Transdermal patches. What's in a brand name? *Nursing 98, 28*(5), 58–59.

Gloth, F.M. (1996). Concerns with chronic analgesic therapy in elderly patients. *American Journal of Medicine, 101*(Suppl. 1A), 19S–24S.

Gorman, C. (1998, July 13). Aspirin without ulcers. *Time*, p. 73.

Harkins, W.W., Kwentus, H., & Price, D. (1990). Pain and suffering in the elderly. In J.J. Bonica (Ed.), *The management of pain* (2nd ed.) (pp. 112–116). Philadelphia: Lea & Febiger.

Hewitt, D., & Foley, K.M. (1996). Pain and pain management. In C. Cassell, H. Cohen, & E. Larson (Eds.), *Geriatric medicine* (3rd ed.) (pp. 865–882). New York: Springer-Verlag.

Hines, C. (1995). Ouchless procedures. *Image, 14*(3), 5–6.

Horgas, A.L., & Tsai, P. (1998). Analgesic drug prescription and use in cognitively impaired nursing home residents. *Nursing Research, 47*, 235–242.

Jacox, A., Carr, D., Payne, R., et al. (1994). *Management of cancer pain. Clinical practice guideline #9.* Rockville, MD: Agency for Health Care Policy and Research, U.S. Department of Health and Human Services, Public Health Service.

Johnson, B.W., & Parris, W.C.V. (1997). Mechanisms of cancer pain. In W.C.V. Parris (Ed.), *Cancer pain management: Principles and practice* (pp. 31–38). Boston: Butterworth-Heinemann.

Karnofsky, D., Abelman, W., & Craver, L. (1948). The use of the nitrogen mustards in the palliative treatment of cancer. *Cancer, 1,* 634.

Kelly, J., & Payne, R. (1993). Pain management in the elderly. In L. Barclay (Ed.), *Clinical geriatric neurology* (pp. 408–423). Philadelphia: Lea & Febiger.

Kingdon, R.T., Stanley, K.J., & Kizior, R.J. (1998). *Handbook for pain management.* Philadelphia: Saunders.

Kozier, B., Erb, G., Blais, K., & Wilkinson, J. (1995). Comfort and pain. In B. Koxier, G. Erb, K. Blais, & J. Wilkinson (Eds.), *Fundamentals of nursing* (pp. 975–1012). New York: Addison-Wesley.

Kurman, M.R. (1993). Systemic therapy (chemotherapy) in the palliative treatment of cancer pain. In R.B. Patt (Ed.), *Cancer pain* (pp. 251–274). Philadelphia: Lippincott.

Lueckenotte, A. (1996). *Gerontological nursing.* St. Louis: Mosby.

Luggen, A.S. (1997). NGNA's strategic plan: Report on Delphi Survey. *Geriatric Nursing, 18*(1), 33–37.

Manfredi, P., Weinstein, S., Chandler, S., & Payne, R. (1997). Comprehensive, medical management: Opioid analgesic. In W.C.V. Parris (Ed.), *Cancer pain management* (pp. 49–68). Boston: Butterworth-Heineman.

McCrae, R. (1984). Situational determinants of coping responses: Loss, threat and challenge. *Journal of Personality and Social Psychology, 46,* 919–928.

Melzack, R. (1975). McGill Pain Questionnaire: Major properties and scoring methods. *Pain, 1,* 357.

Melzack, R. (1992). Phantom limbs. *Scientific American, 266*(4), 120–126.

Miaskowski, C. (1997). How to state your pain. *Coping, 11*(4), 35–36.

Millard, R.W. (1993). Behavior assessment of pain and behavioral pain management. In R.B. Patt (Ed.), *Cancer pain* (pp. 83–97). Philadelphia: Lippincott.

Mor, V., Geer, D.S., & Kastenbaum, R. (Eds.). (1988). *The hospice experiment.* Baltimore: Johns Hopkins University Press.

Morris, J.N., Mor, V., Goldberg, R.J., Sherwood, S., Greer, D.S., & Harris, J. (1986). The effect of treatment setting and patient characteristics on pain in terminal cancer patients: A report for the National Hospice Study. *Journal of Chronic Diseases, 39*(1), 27–35.

Parmalee, P.A., Katz, I.R., & Lawton, M.P. (1991). The relationship of pain to depression among institutionalized aged. *Journal of Gerontology, 46,* 15–21.

Parmalee, P.A, Smith, B., & Katz, I.R. (1993). Pain complaints and cognitive status among elderly institutionalized residents. *Journal of the American Geriatrics Society, 41,* 517–522.

Patt, R.B. (1993a). Classification of cancer pain and cancer pain syndromes. In R.B. Patt (Ed.), *Cancer pain* (pp. 3–22). Philadelphia: Lippincott.

Patt, R.B. (1993b). Peripheral neurolysis and management of cancer pain. In R.B. Patt (Ed.), *Cancer pain* (pp. 359–376). Philadelphia: Lippincott.

Patt, R.B., & Jain, S. (1993). Therapeutic decision making for invasive procedures. In R.B. Patt (Ed.), *Cancer pain* (pp. 275–284). Philadelphia: Lippincott.

Raj, P.P. (1993). Local anesthetic blockade. In R.B. Patt (Ed.), *Cancer pain* (pp. 329–341). Philadelphia: Lippincott.

Rosier, R. (1993). Orthopedic management of cancer pain. In R.B. Patt (Ed.), *Cancer pain* (pp. 461–468). Philadelphia: Lippincott.

Roy, R., & Thomas, M.R. (1987). Elderly persons with pain: A comparative study. *Clinical Journal of Pain, 3,* 513–516.

Skobel, S.W. (1996). Epidural narcotic administration: What nurses should know. *Oncology Nursing Forum, 23,* 1555–1562.

Stein, W. (1996). Cancer pain in the elderly. In B.R. Ferrell & B.A. Ferrell (Eds.), *Pain in the elderly* (pp. 69–80). Seattle: IASP Press.

Stein, W. (1997b). Pain management in long term care facilities. *Clinical Geriatrics, Suppl. 3,* 24–55.

Stein, W., & Ferrell, B.A. (1996). Pain in the nursing home. *Clinics in Geriatric Medicine, 12,* 601–613.

Stein, W., & Miech, R. (1993). Cancer pain in the elderly hospice patient. *Journal of Pain and Symptom Management, 8,* 474–482.

Sternbach, R.R. (1986). Survey of pain in the U.S.: The Nuprin pain report. *Clinical Journal of Pain, 2,* 43–53.

Vallerand, A. (1995). Gender differences in pain. *Image, 27,* 235.

Vanegas, G. (1998). Side effects of morphine administration in cancer patients. *Cancer Nursing, 21,* 289–297.

Ventafridda, V., Tamburini, M., Caraceni, A., DeConno, F., & Naldi, F. (1987). A validation study of the WHO method for cancer pain relief. *Cancer, 59,* 850–856.

Waldman, S., Leak, D., Kennedy, L., & Patt, R. (1993). Intraspinal opioid therapy. In R.B. Patt (Ed.), *Cancer pain.* (pp. 285–302) Philadelphia: Lippincott.

World Health Organization. (1990). *Cancer relief and palliative care. Report of a WHO expert committee.* Geneva, Switzerland: Author.

Zubrod, C., Schneiderman, M., & Frei, E. (1960). Appraisal of methods for the study of chemotherapy in man: Comparative therapeutic trial of nitrogen mustard and triethylene throphospharamide. *Journal of Chronic Diseases, 11,* 7.

Chapter Ten

Symptom Management in the Older Adult With Cancer

Terri Maxwell, RN, MSN, AOCN®
Jacquelynn Nelson, RN, MSN, NP, C, AOCN®

Introduction

Symptom management relates to the care and treatment of side effects that occur as a result of cancer and its progression or as a result of therapy directed toward stabilization or cure. Some treatments produce symptoms that are acute. When side effects from therapies become too severe to tolerate, treatments may need to be stopped, even if the prognosis is affected adversely. Nursing care of the patient and family is essential throughout the cancer experience. This chapter will present several of the most common side effects associated with cancer and its treatment. Specific side effects will be defined and discussed, and the management of therapeutic interventions will be presented.

Nausea and Vomiting

Definition and Description

Nausea and vomiting is one of the most feared consequences of cancer and its treatment. Nausea, retching, and vomiting are separate yet related processes. Nausea is a subjective phenomenon that is manifested by the sensation of the need to vomit. Nausea is described as an uncomfortable wave-like sensation that begins in the back of the throat or abdomen. It often is accompanied by other symptoms mediated by the autonomic nervous system, including tachycardia, perspiration, dizziness, and increased salivation. Retching is the rhythmic and spasmodic contraction of the diaphragm and abdomen. As positive pressure develops, vomiting occurs. Vomiting is the forceful expulsion of stomach or small intestinal contents through the mouth and nose. The vomiting reflex is thought to be a protective mechanism that guards against the ingestion of possible toxic substances.

Occurrence

Despite the use of antiemetics, nausea and vomiting occurs in more than 50% of patients during treatment and in more than 50% of patients during palliative stages (Wickham, 1996). Nausea occurs more frequently than vomiting but is harder to quantify because of its subjective nature. Fortunately, a greater understanding of the pathophysiology of chemotherapy-induced emesis has led to better control of this unpleasant condition. Another recent advance in this area is an improved understanding of the emetic potential of chemotherapy agents. Additionally, the use of combination antiemetics to increase effectiveness and decrease toxicity and the development of a highly effective class of antiemetics called "selective serotonin antagonists" have proven to be beneficial. Prompt management is imperative because of the stress and the potentially life-threatening dehydration sometimes caused by nausea and vomiting.

Pathophysiology of Emesis

Nausea and vomiting is a complex physiologic process with a mechanism that is still not completely understood. Vomiting involves the gastrointestinal system, the brain, and a variety of neurotransmitters. Vomiting is controlled by the vomiting center (VC), which is located in the area of the lateral reticular formulation of the fourth ventricle in the medulla. The VC is activated by the following afferent pathways (Violette, 1998).
- Vagal visceral afferent associated with gastric irritation
- Sympathetic visceral afferent stimulated by irritation
- Ischemia or obstruction of chest or abdominal organs
- Vestibulocerebellar afferent involving the inner ear
- Midbrain afferent related to increased intracranial pressure
- Cerebral cortex and limbic system afferent responding to sensory input such as sight and smell

Chemotherapy-Induced Emesis

Chemotherapy-induced emesis associated with agents such as cisplatin is thought to be mediated by stimulation of receptors in the central nervous system (CNS) and gastrointestinal tract. The primary mechanism of cisplatin-induced emesis is via vagal afferent under serotonergic control. Serotonin ($5-HT_3$) is released from enterochromaffin cells located in the lining of the small intestine in response to chemotherapy-induced cell damage, which activates $5-HT_3$ receptors on vagal and splanchnic nerves. This, in turn, activates the chemoreceptor trigger zone (CTZ) located adjacent to the postrema. The CTZ, rich in both $5-HT_3$ and dopamine receptors, responds directly to chemical toxins and neurotransmitters carried by blood and cerebral spinal fluid (Allan, 1992). Vomiting results when the CTZ stimulates the VC. Effective antiemetics have been developed in response to an improved understanding of the complex neurotransmitter role in chemotherapy-induced emesis.

Miscellaneous Factors

In addition to VC stimulation caused by toxins (either disease- or treatment-related), a number of other factors can induce nausea and vomiting in patients with cancer. Common causes include irritation or obstruction of the gastrointestinal tract, including biliary obstruction, peptic ulceration, gastric compression, bowel obstruction, delayed gastric emptying, esophagitis, and constipation. Liver failure, medications such as opioids and antibiotics, severe cough, and CNS disease all may cause significant nausea and vomiting. An array of psychological factors, including anxiety, depression, sights, smells, and tastes, also have been implicated.

Classification of Emesis

Chemotherapy-induced emesis has been classified as the following.
- Acute: Nausea and vomiting that occurs within the first 24 hours after chemotherapy
- Delayed: Nausea and vomiting that persists or develops 24 hours after chemotherapy
- Anticipatory: Nausea and vomiting that occurs as a conditioned response to stimuli such as chemotherapy
- Refractory: Nausea and vomiting that is resistant or nonresponsive to treatment.

Acute Chemotherapy-Induced Nausea and Vomiting

Acute chemotherapy-induced nausea and vomiting is best controlled by using appropriate antiemetic therapy prophylactically. If nausea and vomiting is not controlled adequately during the first 24-hour period, anticipatory as well as delayed nausea and vomiting may accompany subsequent treatment.

Delayed Nausea and Vomiting

Delayed nausea and vomiting may last up to seven days, peaking at 48–72 hours. Figure 10.1 lists drugs associated with delayed nausea and vomiting. The mechanisms underlying this condition are not well defined but are believed to be related to the release of dopamine, decreased gastrointestinal motility, and the release of cellular breakdown products.

Anticipatory Nausea and Vomiting

Anticipatory nausea and vomiting is a classic Pavlovian response experienced by patients who have had difficulty with nausea and vomiting after prior chemotherapy. Anticipatory nausea can occur without actual vomiting (Wickham, 1996). The best treatment for anticipatory nausea and vomiting is to prevent nausea after the initial chemotherapy course. Once established, it is difficult to eradicate. Other interventions include behavioral interventions and the administration of anxiolytics such as lorazepam.

Consequences of excessive vomiting include dehydration, weight loss, malnutrition, esophageal tears, aspiration pneumonia, and decreased quality of life with depression, anxiety, and distress (Jenns, 1994). If nausea and vomiting is too distressing, patients may delay or refuse further courses of potentially curative or palliative chemotherapy.

Nausea and Vomiting in the Older Adult

Age-related changes, as described by Ebersole and Hess (1998), that affect the gastrointestinal system can cause a decrease in gastrointestinal muscle strength and motility, resulting in decreased peristalsis. In the stomach, there are fewer cells responsible for secreting hydrochloric acid and pepsin is decreased. Gastric irritation is more prevalent as the stomach pH increases and the protective

Figure 10.1. Drugs Associated With Delayed Nausea and Vomiting

• High-dose cisplatin	• Doxorubicin
• Cyclophosphamide	• Carboplatin
• Mitomycin	

alkaline mucus of the stomach is lost. In addition, gastric emptying time is increased as smooth muscle is lost during the aging process.

A common perception exists that elderly patients tolerate chemotherapy more poorly than younger patients do and have a higher rate of chemotherapy-related side effects. To the contrary, Dodd, Onishki, Dibble, and Larson (1996) measured differences in nausea, vomiting, and retching between younger and older (> 65 years) outpatients receiving chemotherapy and found that younger patients had consistently (although statistically insignificant) higher nausea and vomiting scores despite similar levels of aggressiveness of chemotherapy agents. In a prospective study of terminally ill hospice patients, Reuben and Mor (1986) also demonstrated that younger patients had higher rates of nausea and vomiting independent of chemotherapy.

Assessment

When assessing nausea and vomiting, a number of parameters need to be examined. A careful history and physical may reveal a variety of information that places patients at increased risk for nausea and vomiting, including hepatomegaly, dehydration, obstructive symptoms, CNS disease, and psychological distress. Patients at high risk for severe vomiting related to chemotherapy include those with high trait anxiety, a history of motion sickness, food allergies, and food aversions; those who expect to be sick; and younger patients (Dodd et al., 1996).

No comprehensive tool exists that can accurately and simply measure nausea and vomiting. Patient report is still the most effective means of assessing nausea (see Figure 10.2). In the hospital, intake and output records may help to indicate fluid volume deficits. Patient weight is an accurate and easy-to-record tool for use in assessing fluid or body mass losses or gains. Persistent symptoms may require further diagnostic workup, including but not limited to endoscopy, colonoscopy, barium radiography, and computerized tomography (CT) scans of the abdomen and brain.

Treatment

Treatment of nausea and vomiting depends, in a large part, on the presumed underlying cause. Treatment may be directed at correcting the underlying disease or condition leading to the nausea and vomiting or alleviating the symptoms with a pharmacologic approach.

Pharmacologic Treatments

Pharmacologic interventions include several classifications of antiemetics, each with its own mechanism of action and associated side effects. A brief review of antiemetics commonly used to treat patients with cancer follows. Table 10.1 also presents a list of commonly used antiemetics.

Figure 10.2. Assessment of Nausea and Vomiting

- Does vomiting accompany nausea?
- What factors stimulate nausea (e.g., odors, medication, activity)?
- Is your nausea associated with eating?
- Does anything relieve the nausea and vomiting?
- Are you able to keep down any solids or liquids?
- Does anything relieve the nausea and vomiting?
- What other symptoms do you have (e.g., headache, dizziness, heartburn, constipation)?

Table 10.1. Commonly Used Drugs for Chemotherapy-Induced Emesis

Drug	Route	Dose	Schedule	Side Effects
Prochlorperazine	PO	5–10 mg	4–6 h	Sedation
	IM, IV	5–14 mg	3–6 h	Extrapyramidal reactions
	PR	25 mg	8–12 h	Anticholinergic
Metoclopramide	PO	1–3 mg/kg or 10–40 mg	2–6 h	Extrapyramidal reactions Sedation
	IV	1–3 mg/kg	4–6 h	Diarrhea
Dexamethasone	PO	4–8 mg	2–4 times/ day before chemotherapy then every 4–6 h	Increased appetite Mood changes Psychosis Insomnia
	IV	10–20 mg		
Lorazepam	PO	1–3 mg	4–6 h	Sedation
	IV	1–1.5 mg/ml	4–6 h	Confusion Amnesia
Ondansetron	PO	8 mg TID 32 mg	30 minutes prior to chemotherapy x 1	Headache Diarrhea Constipation Sedation
Granisetron	PO	1–2 mg 10 mcg/kg or 1 mg	30 minutes prior to chemotherapy	See Ondansetron
Dolasetron mesylate	PO	1 mg	30 minutes prior to chemotherapy	See Ondansetron
	IV	1 mg		

Phenothiazine Agents

Phenothiazines were the first class of antiemetics developed and are believed to exert their effect through dopamine blockade. They are used with mild to moderately emetic chemotherapy agents and as general-purpose antiemetics. Phenothiazines are available in multiple preparations, including parenteral, oral, and rectal suppository forms. Two commonly used phenothiazines are prochlorperazine (Compazine®, SmithKline Beecham Pharmaceuticals, Philadelphia, PA) and chlorpromazine (Thorazine®, SmithKline Beecham Pharmaceuticals). Side effects include sedation, akathisia, hypotension, and dystonic reactions. Prochlorperazine is useful for some patients who experience radiation-induced nausea or delayed nausea and vomiting after chemotherapy.

Butyrophenone Agents

Butyrophenone agents, which include haloperidol (Haldol®, Ortho-McNeil Pharmaceutical, Raritan, NJ) and droperidol are less frequently used. Haloperidol is associated with a greater incidence of Parkinson's-like symptoms and is reserved for use mainly with terminally ill patients (Allan, 1992).

Procainamide Derivatives

Metoclopramide (Reglan®, A.H. Robbins Company, Richmond, VA) is a procainamide derivative with peripheral and central antiemetic action. At high doses, it has $5-HT_3$ blocking activity, as well as dopamine antagonist activity. Metoclopramide also promotes gastric emptying, making it useful for gastric stasis and gastroesophageal reflux (Schuster, 1994). Its use in the treatment of chemotherapy-induced nausea and vomiting has been largely supplanted by more selective serotonin antagonists. Side effects include mild sedation, weakness, restlessness, and diarrhea (Pisters & Kris, 1998). Metoclopramide has been associated with the development of extrapyramidal reactions manifesting as acute dystonias or dyskinesias, although these reactions rarely occur in patients over age 30 (Kris et al., 1983). Parkinsonian effects are more common in older patients (Allan, 1992). Metoclopramide remains a useful agent for treating gastroparesis in doses of 5–10 mg orally two hours before meals. Domperidone is used to treat nausea and vomiting related to Parkinson's disease (Allan). As with metoclopramide, caution should be used because of extrapyramidal reactions.

Corticosteroids

Corticosteroids such as dexamethasone commonly are used to treat nausea and vomiting related to cerebral edema or as adjuncts to prevent chemotherapy-related nausea and vomiting. The mechanism of action is completely unknown, but an antiprostaglandin effect has been postulated.

Cannabinoid Agents

The cannabinoid agent dronabinol (Marinol®, Roxane Laboratories, Columbus, OH) is not recommended as an antiemetic in elderly patients because of its high rate of side effects. Side effects such as sedation, dry mouth, disorientation, and dizziness have been reported in middle-aged and older adults (Pisters & Kris, 1998).

Selective $5-HT_3$ Antagonists

Findings indicating that metoclopramide, in addition to dopamine antagonism, was able to produce a more complete antiemetic effect by blocking the $5-HT_3$ receptor swiftly led to the testing of other selective $5-HT_3$ antagonists. Research suggests that $5-HT_3$ antagonists block radiation- or chemotherapy-induced emesis by competing for the binding of serotonin to the $5-HT_3$ receptors in the wall of the gut and may act at the level of the $5-HT_3$ receptors in the CNS as well. Presently, three drugs in this class are available: ondansetron (Zofran®, Burroughs Wellcome Inc., Research Triangle Park, NC), granisetron (Kytril®, SmithKline Beecham Pharmaceuticals), and dolasetron mesylate (Anzemet®, Hoechst Marion Roussel, Kansas City, MO). To date, no differences have been reported regarding the therapeutic efficacy of the three drugs (Cleri, 1995). They have been found to be safe and well tolerated. Headaches are the most common side effect reported. The selective $5-HT_3$ antagonists are available in both IV and oral preparations. The high cost associated with both the oral and IV forms has limited their use to most emetic chemotherapy regimens or for radiation-induced nausea and vomiting. They are not indicated for delayed nausea and vomiting (Latreille et al., 1998) or as general-purpose antiemetics. However, Mystakidou, Befon, Liossi, and Vlachos (1998) demonstrated that the serotonin antagonist tropisetron (not yet available in the United States), alone or in combination with dexamethasone, was much more effective than the conventional antiemetic regimen of chlorpromazine plus dexamethasone in controlling persistent nausea and vomiting in terminally ill patients. Oral serotonin antagonists are as effective as IV forms, are less costly, and are well suited for home, outpatient, and office use.

Nonpharmacologic Behavioral Approaches

Numerous nonpharmacologic approaches have been used to prevent or treat nausea and vomiting. These include hypnosis, distraction, behavioral modification, relaxation exercises, guided imagery, and deconditioning. These approaches take time and patient motivation but are generally inexpensive and do not have side effects, and they may be helpful adjuncts to pharmacologic therapies.

Summary

Nausea and vomiting, whether caused by treatment or the underlying disease, is one of the most distressing symptoms related to cancer. The advent of new and combination antiemetics has done much to improve nausea and vomiting related to chemotherapy or radiation treatments. Delayed nausea and vomiting remains a challenge that requires further research and the development of effective agents. Elderly patients have a lower incidence of treatment-induced nausea and vomiting but are at higher risk for morbidity if it is not controlled. Nurses have an important role in assessing and managing this difficult symptom.

Constipation

Definition and Description

Constipation is a common and distressing symptom experienced by patients with cancer, especially older adults. Constipation is a subjective term used to describe unsatisfactory bowel movements. The movements may be hard, small, infrequent, and associated with straining. When untreated, constipation can lead to a cycle of distress, resulting in decreased appetite, decreased mobility, and increased pain. Constipation, like pain, is a subjective symptom that cannot be easily quantified.

Pathophysiology

The cause of constipation is multifactorisal and may be related to a patient's age or disease state. Age-related causative factors include reduced colonic motility, inadequate fluid and fiber intake, habitual failure to respond to the urge to defecate, depression, increased stress, environmental changes, and long-term laxative abuse (Yakabowich, 1990). In some cases, elderly patients have poor pelvic floor muscle coordination, diminished contractual muscle tone, and loss of neuronal sensitivity of the bowel.

Cancer-related causes of constipation include the direct effect of tumors associated with colon or pelvic cancers resulting in compression of the large intestine or by disrupting its neuronal mechanism. Metabolic disorders, particularly hypercalcemia and hypokalemia, may contribute to constipation in patients with cancer. Uremia resulting from kidney failure also may induce constipation. Neurologic causes include spinal cord compression and tumor infiltration of the sacral plexus. More commonly, constipation is related to cancer therapy, the use of opioids for pain control, and debilitation associated with advanced disease (Portenoy, 1987).

Nonmalignant causes of constipation include postoperative adhesions, radiation-induced colitis or strictures, and anal fissures or prominent hemorrhoids causing anal pain. Diseases such as diabetes mellitus, Parkinson's disease, and hypothyroidism that may coincide with a malignancy also predispose patients to constipation.

Physiology

To understand constipation and its treatment, an understanding of the mechanism of normal defecation is necessary. Normal colon activity involves mixing and propulsive movements caused by both voluntary and involuntary muscles. Activities such as food ingestion initiate propulsive, peristaltic waves in the colon that propel fecal material toward the rectum (Gross, 1994). Peristalsis is stimulated when the presence of fecal material stretches the bowel wall. The strongest peristaltic waves usually occur following breakfast. When peristalsis becomes sluggish, stool transit time is increased, more fluid than normal is absorbed, and stools become hard, dry, and more difficult to pass.

The urge to defecate occurs when enough stool has collected in the rectum to initiate stretch receptors located in the anus. Sacral nerve segments initiate involuntary internal sphincter contractions followed by voluntary contraction of the external anal sphincter. Contraction of abdominal muscles helps to facilitate bowel emptying. If the urge to defecate is repeatedly ignored, sensitivity of the rectal nerves will be diminished and constipation can ensue. As the stool remains in the rectal vault, more fluid is absorbed, resulting in hard, small stools.

Symptoms

Constipation, like pain, is a subjective symptom that cannot be quantified easily. Symptoms include decreased stool frequency; excessive straining; abdominal cramping or fullness; a sense of incomplete evacuation and tenesmus; increased gas; and abdominal bloating (Cameron, 1992). Patients also may complain of hard, dry stools.

Assessment

A careful history and physical should be performed to help to identify the cause of constipation. A careful review of patients' medications, including over-the-counter medications, should be performed. The physical examination should include a digital rectal exam, careful inspection of the perineal region, and auscultation of the abdomen. Assessment of the abdomen may reveal gaseous distention, decreased bowel sounds in all quadrants, and dull mixed with tympanic sounds (Cameron, 1992).

Patients with new or progressive constipation without apparent etiology will require additional tests. The goal of this evaluation should be to identify treatable causes. Stool should be checked for occult blood. A metabolic evaluation should include renal and hepatic function tests and the measurement of electrolyte levels and thyroid hormone levels. Radiographic evaluation should include plain abdominal films to exclude megacolon or obstruction. A CT scan or ultrasound may be used to evaluate extraluminal pathology. Barium studies or endoscopy can be used to evaluate intraluminal processes and to help to identify sites of extraluminal compression. Magnetic resonance imaging of the spine should be considered if constipation is associated with back pain or lower extremity weakness (Portenoy, 1987).

Management

When treating constipation in elderly patients with cancer, every effort should be made to determine the etiology of the constipation and direct treatment accordingly. Identifying patients at risk for the development of constipation is important because constipation often is easier to prevent than to treat once established. Preventive programs should include exercise, adequate fluid intake, a fiber-rich diet, and laxatives, when necessary. Figure 10.3 presents a nonpharmacologic approach to preventing constipation.

Exercise

Regular exercise stimulates gut motility. Unfortunately, many elderly patients with cancer are immobilized for various reasons, including neuromuscular disorders, arthritis, and generalized weakness and fatigue. A walking program and increased activity are recommended whenever feasible.

Fluid Intake

Liquids are natural stool softeners. The recommended fluid intake is 2,000–3,000 ml per day (Brown & Everett, 1990). Encouraging or assisting patients to drink small amounts of fluids frequently is recommended. Fluids containing caffeine should be avoided because caffeine has a diuretic effect that may decrease body fluids (Yakabowich, 1990).

Fiber

When added to the diet, fiber reduces colon transit time, resulting in improved ease and increased frequency of defecation. Fiber helps to draw water into the stool, making it heavier, softer, and bulkier. The recommended amount of dietary fiber is 6–10 g per day (Yakabowich, 1990). When bran is added as a bulking agent, the recommended daily supplemental dosage is 2–4 g initially (Brown & Everett, 1990). This amount may be increased up to 10 g as tolerated. Prunes add 2 g of fiber, but prune juice has almost no fiber (Yakabowich). Fiber content should be decreased if bloating or cramping occurs.

Numerous studies have documented that high-fiber diets with a controlled fluid intake effectively reduce laxative use and assist in controlling constipation among long-term care residents. Beverly and Travis (1992) found that a natural laxative mixture added to the diet of elderly psychogeriatric patients managed constipation as successfully as other bowel methods, including a bowel protocol with laxative administration, suppositories, or sodium biphosphate lactulose enemas. Approximately half of this special population had bowel movements two to three times per week. The need for enemas and suppositories was greatly reduced, and significant cost savings occurred (Beverly & Travis). A program of increased fluid and dietary fiber in a chronic-care hospital resulted in not only less constipation and less reliance on laxatives but also in improved mental status functioning and decreased episodes of confusion among patients (Benton, O'Hara, Chen, Harper, & Johnston, 1997).

A variety of natural laxative mixtures have been proposed (Beverly & Travis, 1992; Brown & Everett, 1990). Figure 10.4 lists natural preparations that prevent or manage constipation. A high-fiber approach is contraindicated

Figure 10.3. Nonpharmacologic Measures to Prevent Constipation

- Increase fluid intake.
- Increase fiber, fruit juice, and fruit.
- Provide privacy and timely toileting habits.
- Modify medications when possible.
- Encourage regular activity.

Figure 10.4. Natural Constipation-Prevention Remedies

Natural Laxative Recipe	Fiber Supplement Recipe
1 lb raisins 1 lb currants 1 lb prunes 1 lb figs 1 lb dates 1 28-ounce container undiluted prune concentrate Put fruit through a grinder. Mix with prune concentrate in large mixer (mixture will be very thick). Store in large-mouthed plastic container. Refrigerate. Take 30 ml twice a day if constipated.	Combine 2 cups Kellogg's All Bran® cereal 2 cups applesauce 1 cup 100% prune juice Start with 1 ounce per day, increasing to 2 ounces as needed. Store in refrigerator. A minimum of 1,500 ml/day of fluids is essential.
Note. Based on information from Beverly & Travis, 1992.	*Note.* Based on information from Brown & Everett, 1990.

in patients at risk for obstruction and in patients with advanced disease and motility disturbances that are too severe to allow for free passage of bulky stool through the colon (Portenoy, 1987).

Laxative Management

In elderly patients with cancer, laxatives generally need to be employed because many patients are either unable to alter their diet and activity levels or have such refractory constipation that lifestyle changes alone are not adequate to rectify the problem. The decision about which laxative to prescribe is based on a working knowledge of the pharmacology, anticipated effects, and potential toxicity of each laxative (Portenoy, 1987).

Bulk-Forming Laxatives

Bulk-forming laxatives include bran, psyllium (Metamucil®, Procter & Gamble, Cincinnati, OH), and methylcellulose (Citrucel®, SmithKline Beecham). These agents are useful for elderly patients with diminished colonic response. They are composed of indigestible fibers that pass through the stomach and increase stool bulk and soften stool by increasing mass and water content. Eight to 10 eight-ounce glasses of fluid per day help to prevent clumping of bulk laxatives and to promote soft stools. They should not be given concomitantly with drugs such as digoxin or aspirin because they may inhibit their absorption (Yakabowich, 1990). Furthermore, Metamucil contains 200 mg of sodium per pack. Citrucel is less gritty than Metamucil and contains no sodium but does contain 5 g of sugar per dose (Yakabowich). No studies have examined the efficacy of or dosing requirements for bulk-forming laxatives, and these agents are contraindicated in patients with bowel obstruction. They generally are not considered to be effective or feasible for use in patients with advanced cancer.

Osmotic Laxatives

Osmotic (saline) laxatives include magnesium salts, sodium salts, and lactulose. They act by osmotically drawing water into the lumen of the large intestine, thereby increasing bulk and stimulating peristalsis. Saline cathartics are thought to inhibit fluid and electrolyte absorption from the jejunum and ileum. They usually produce a stool within two to six hours. Sulfate and magnesium salts are considered to be the most potent of this group, and magnesium salts are the most commonly used. Saline cathartics are contraindicated in patients with renal dysfunction because the sodium and other minerals can accumulate. Sodium salts may be problematic in patients with congestive heart disease. Osmotic laxatives require fluid replacement to prevent dehydration.

Lactulose, an osmotic agent, is a synthesized disaccharide that passes through the intestine unabsorbed. It eventually is degraded by bacteria in the colon to short chain organic acids that act as osmotic agents. The net effect is the accumulation of fluid in the colon and the production of a soft stool. A number of studies have shown lactulose to be effective in treating geriatric patients (Beverly & Travis, 1992). Tolerance did not develop, and fecal impaction rates decreased. Anecdotally, lactulose is the laxative of choice for advanced cancer after senna (Senokot S®, The Purdue Frederick Company, Norwalk, CT) is no longer effective. Side effects include flatulence, cramping, diarrhea, and electrolyte imbalances. It should be used with caution in diabetic patients because of its sugar content. Lactulose is expensive but may be covered by prescription plans.

Stool Softeners

Surfactants comprise the class of laxatives commonly referred to as "stool softeners." These agents, known as docusates, have a detergent effect that allows water to penetrate hard stools. The two most commonly used agents in this class are docusate sodium (Colace®, Roberts, Eatontown, NJ), which is a sodium salt, and docusate calcium (Surfak®, Upjohn Company, Kalamazoo, MI), which is a calcium salt. They often are used in combination with other cathartics such as senna, although no controlled studies have established their efficacy (Portenoy, 1987). Docusate has been shown to be ineffective in altering the incidence of constipation among elderly medical patients (Gross, 1994).

Stimulant Laxatives

Stimulant (contact) laxatives are perhaps the most commonly used drugs to treat constipation. There are three basic types: castor oil, anthraquinones (senna and cascara), and bisacodyl (Dulcolax®, Novartis Consumer Health, Inc., Summit, NJ). Castor oil is not recommended because its violent cathartic action is difficult to control (Levy, 1992).

Anthraquinones act primarily in the colon after coming into contact with colonic bacteria. They are thought to work by inducing peristalsis and by inhibiting water absorption in the small and large intestine (Mercandante, 1998). They tend to have a mild laxative effect but may cause cramping at higher doses. Senna is effective in treating or preventing opioid-induced constipation. Its onset of action is 6–10 hours. Cascara, often used in combination with milk of magnesia, is generally mild and well-tolerated.

Diphenylmethanes include bisacodyl (Dulcolax) and phenolphthalein. Phenolphthalein is found in many over-the-counter laxative preparations, including Feen-a-Mint® (Schering-Plough, Madison, NJ), Ex-Lax® (Novartis Consumer Health, Inc.), and Correctol® (Schering-Plough). Phenolphthalein's laxative effect often is difficult to predict and control and may last for several days. Toxic reactions include cramping, diarrhea, skin reactions, photosensitivity, and hypersensitivity-type encephalitis (Levy, 1992). Bisacodyl has no reported systemic toxicity and is preferred in elderly patients. When bisacodyl is taken orally, a bowel movement usually is produced within 6 hours (8 to 12 hours if taken at bedtime). It comes in a 5 mg tablet and a 10 mg suppository. The tablets are enteric coated to avoid release in the stomach, where they can irritate the gastric mucosa. They should not be taken within one hour of antacids or H_2 blockers to prevent dissolution of the enteric coating (Yakabowich, 1990). Bisacodyl's stimulating effect may be quite strong, but it is often a good choice for refractory, narcotic-induced constipation.

Lubricant Laxatives

Mineral oil belongs to the lubricant (emollient) laxative group. Mineral oil produces a soft stool by lubricating fecal contents. Mineral oil is used infrequently and not recommended because of potentially serious and unpleasant adverse effects. Aspiration of mineral oil may cause lipid pneumonia, especially in debilitated or bedridden patients. In large doses, it may cause seepage from the rectum, resulting in soiled linens or bed clothes.

Suppositories

Suppositories act mechanically to stimulate sensory receptors in the rectum to initiate defecation. Glycerin suppositories act not only mechanically but also draw fluid into the rectum. They work well for elderly patients experiencing infrequent constipation. Frequent use may result in rectal irritation. Bisacodyl is available in suppository form and takes effect in 15–60 minutes. Bisacodyl suppositories may cause cramping, rectal urgency, and a mild burning sensation. Suppositories require less nursing time than enemas and generally are more acceptable to patients. They are not very effective if hard, dry stool is present.

Enemas

Enemas, consisting of tap water, saline, or soap suds, stimulate the bowel by mechanically distending the colon and stimulating rectal wall nerves to initiate peristalsis. They are used to evacuate the distal colon. Incorrect use can result in fluid and electrolyte imbalances and, in rare cases, colonic perforation (Yakabowich, 1990). Very thin or frail older patients may require smaller fluid volumes when receiving irrigating enemas. Too much fluid may induce shock. The fluid should be warmed to improve patient comfort. Enemas are contraindicated after recent colon or rectal surgery or myocardial infarction.

Miscellaneous Agents

Other drugs useful in treating constipation include metoclopramide (Reglan®, A.H. Robins Company, Richmond, VA) and cisapride (Propulsid®, Janssen Pharmaceutica, Titusville, NJ). Both are prokinetic agents that stimulate gastric emptying and accelerate small bowel transit (Levy, 1992). Propulsid may be safer to use with elderly patients because it lacks the antidopaminergic effects associated with Reglan.

Choice of Laxative

Figure 10.5 presents an example of a bowel protocol. Before starting a laxative, treat underlying causes whenever possible and discontinue nonessential constipation drugs when feasible. Make available bedside commodes for patients who are less ambulatory, and provide privacy whenever possible.

When employing laxatives, bulk agents alone often result in a large collection of soft stool that patients are unable to pass. For that reason, mild stimulants in addition to bulk agents often are used. An osmotic agent such as milk of magnesia is another alternative. Additionally, a combination of a stimulant and stool softener might be helpful. Stool softener preparations are especially useful in patients with hard, difficult-to-pass stools and those with anal fissures or hemorrhoids. Patients with hypotonic constipation should not use stool softeners alone because

Figure 10.5. Proposed Bowel Regimen for Older Patients With Cancer

Begin with a stool softener and gentle laxative.
- Senokot S, one to two tablets two to three times/day

If no bowel movement occurs within 48 hours, ADD ONE:
- Milk of magnesia
- Dulcolax tablet, 5 mg, one to two tablets

If no bowel movement occurs within 72 hours, TRY ONE:
- Dulcolax suppository, 10 mg
- Magnesium citrate, 8 ounces
- Fleet enema

Administer oral naloxone hydrochloride for refractory opioid-induced constipation.

the soft stool will be difficult to expel. If stool is present in the rectum, a suppository or enema may be helpful. Laxatives should be used prophylactically in high-risk patients, especially in those on opioids, because constipation is easier to prevent than to treat. Such an approach undoubtedly will help to improve quality of life for elderly patients with advanced cancer.

Opioid-Induced Constipation

Constipation, the most common side effect of opioid analgesics, occurs as a result of the opioid binding to the gastrointestinal tract, leading to decreased peristalsis, reduced intestinal secretions, and increased resorption of fluids from the colon. A bowel regimen must be initiated in people who will be maintained on chronic opioid therapy. Dietary modifications and bulk laxatives alone rarely are adequate for this group of patients (Levy, 1992). Although the optimal laxative for patients has not been empirically determined, anecdotal reports indicate that senna (Senokot) is the drug of choice. One Senokot tablet reverses the constipating effect of 120 mg of codeine (Levy, 1992). In a study comparing the efficacy of senna to that of lactulose, Agra, Sacristran, Gonzalez, Portuques, and Calvo (1998) found no differences related to efficacy or adverse effects but recommended the use of senna because of its lower cost. Oral naloxone has been found to reverse opioid-induced constipation without precipitating withdrawal symptoms or a return of pain in opioid-dependent patients (Culpepper-Morgan et al., 1992; Sykes, 1996). The recommended dose of naloxone is 2–4 ampules orally every two hours to a maximum of 15 ampules (Sykes). In refractory patients, 100 mcg of Cytotec® (Searle, Chicago, IL) and 20 mg of Propulsid can be added.

Some opioids are less constipating than others and may be selected for this purpose. Chronic administration of codeine should be avoided because of its severe constipating side effect. Transdermal fentanyl patches are associated with significantly less constipation when compared to sustained-relief oral morphine (Ahmedzai & Brooks, 1997).

Fecal Impaction

Fecal impaction occurs when a hard, dry mass of stool becomes lodged in the rectum or sigmoid colon. Fecal impaction is a common cause of fecal incontinence in older people. Paradoxical diarrhea occurs when watery stool is passed around the mass of hard stool. The clinical characteristics of fecal incontinence secondary to fecal impaction are liquid or semisolid stool soiling many times a day (Brocklehurst, 1992). Fecal impaction may result from inadequate fluid intake, poor bowel habits, dehydration, inactivity, and constipating drugs such as opioids.

Fecal impaction requires digital removal when enemas, suppositories, and laxatives are unsuccessful. Because of the discomfort associated with impaction removal, patients should be premedicated with an analgesic such as subcutaneous morphine prior to the procedure. Manual disimpaction is contraindicated in neutropenic patients. In most cases, disimpaction should be followed with oral laxatives to clear the colon. Once the impacted feces have been removed, a laxative regimen should be used to prevent the condition from recurring.

Summary

Constipation is a very common malady in elderly patients with cancer. It has many etiologies in this population. Assessment of high-risk individuals and management with lifestyle alterations and laxative regimens are imperative. Prevention of constipation in elderly patients with cancer should be the ultimate goal.

Diarrhea

Definition and Description

Diarrhea exists when one of the following is present: abnormal increase in daily stool weight, increase in water content, or increase in frequency of stools. It is accompanied by urgency, perianal discomfort, and incontinence (Mercandante, 1998). Diarrhea results when the balance among absorption, secretion, and intestinal motility is disrupted. Its consequences may be severe, including dehydration, electrolyte imbalances, malabsorption, and skin breakdown. Quality of life also may be affected, resulting in emotional and physical discomfort (Hogan, 1998).

Occurrence

Diarrhea is a common occurrence in patients with cancer. An estimated 10% of patients in the United States who have advanced cancer will experience diarrhea (Levy, 1992). Diarrhea can be classified as acute (i.e., lasting less than two weeks) or chronic (i.e., lasting more than two weeks).

Pathophysiology

Diarrhea commonly is classified by type according to characteristics. Different types of diarrhea include osmotic, secretory, motility-associated, and exudative.

Characteristics of osmotic diarrhea include the presence of large volumes of fluid and electrolytes that overwhelm the capacity of the bowel (Rutledge & Engelking, 1998). It usually is caused by the ingestion of nonabsorbable substances that are hyperosmolar and is characterized by large volumes of watery stool. Examples of such substances are sorbitol, citrates, lactulose, and enteral feeding solutions (Engelking, 1998). The hallmark sign of osmotic diarrhea is that it resolves when patients fast or the causative agent is withdrawn (Martz, 1996).

Secretory diarrhea is stimulated by outside agents that affect intestinal transportation of water. This results in the accumulation of intestinal fluid. It is usually caused by endocrine-secreting tumors or pathogens such as *Clostridium difficile* (*C. difficile*). Secretory diarrhea is manifested by large volumes of watery stool that persist despite fasting (Rutledge & Engelking, 1998).

Motility-associated diarrhea results in rapid transit of stool related to neural stimuli. It is described as frequent, small, semisolid stools. Motility-associated diarrhea can result from such disorders as irritable bowel syndrome, narcotic withdrawal, peristaltic stimulants, stress, anxiety, and fear.

Exudative diarrhea is caused by the discharge of mucus, serum proteins, and blood into the bowel lumen, resulting in bowel inflammation or ulceration. This type of diarrhea frequently is caused by and is a direct result of damage to the bowel mucosa caused by external beam radiation therapy.

Etiology

The causes of cancer-related diarrhea are multifactorial. Many older adults suffer from concomitant illnesses in addition to cancer. Gastrointestinal disorders such as diverticulitis, irritable bowel syndrome, and constipation with associated laxative use can lead to diarrhea. Older adults also take many oral medications to control illnesses such as diabetes mellitus, hypertension, and heart disease, which also may alter bowel motility.

Diarrhea Caused by Tumors

Certain types of neuro-endocrine tumors (e.g., carcinoid, VIPoma, gastrinoma) directly can cause diarrhea (Hogan, 1998). These tumors secrete polypeptides and hormones, which results in profuse secretory diarrhea by interfering with the function of digestive enzymes, damaging mucosa, and increasing motility.

Chemotherapy-Associated Diarrhea

Many types of chemotherapy, particularly antimetabolites such as fluorouracil, cause diarrhea. Chemotherapy exerts its effects on the most rapidly dividing cells in the body. These cells consist not only of tumor cells but also of normal cells that line the gastrointestinal tract. This results in inflammation of the bowel wall, causing damage to the intestinal villi. Subsequently, decreased absorption leads to increased secretion of intestinal fluids and electrolytes, resulting in profuse secretory diarrhea (Mercandante, 1995).

Irinotecan has been noted for its early and late diarrhea syndromes. The incidence of irinotecan-induced diarrhea has been reported to be as high as 50%–80% (Wadler et al., 1998). The early diarrhea is actually a cholinergic reaction and is easily reversed with atropine. The late diarrhea needs to be addressed immediately, and antidiarrheals need to be aggressively instituted to prevent severe episodes with resultant dehydration and electrolyte imbalances. Figure 10.6 lists common chemotherapeutic agents associated with diarrhea.

Diarrhea also is prevalent in patients with graft-versus-host disease after bone marrow transplantation. This diarrhea is secretory in nature and occurs secondary to an immune reaction that attacks the cells that line the gastrointestinal tract, causing cell necrosis (Ippoliti & Neumann, 1998).

Radiation-Induced Diarrhea

Radiation therapy that encompasses the intestines can result in diarrhea. The diarrhea usually is dose-dependent and occurs with doses from 1,500–3,000 cGy (Martz, 1996). Chronic ischemic enteritis can be a late effect of radiation therapy that results from vascular damage to the bowel wall. This can lead to

Figure 10.6. Chemotherapy Drugs Associated With Diarrhea

- Fluorouracil
- Irinotecan
- Methotrexate
- Thioguanine
- Doxorubicin
- Nitrosoureas
- Paclitaxel
- Cisplatin
- Hydroxyurea

absorption problems, stricture, obstruction, fistula formation, and proctitis associated with chronic bloody stools (Martz).

C. Difficile Diarrhea

Pseudomembranous enterocolitis resulting from C. *difficile* infection is a common cause of diarrhea in patients with cancer who have been treated with antibiotics or chemotherapy. C. *difficile* infection can lead to severe hypovolemia, dehydration, perforation, and hemorrhage if left untreated (Martz, 1996).

Other Causes of Diarrhea

Other causes of cancer-related diarrhea include gastrostomy tube feedings secondary to a cancer-related problem; gastrointestinal surgical procedures such as bowel resection resulting in dumping syndrome; disease-related stress; fecal impaction; medications; and diet (Abbasi, 1998).

Clinical Manifestations

Diarrhea can result in a multitude of clinical manifestations and can be life-threatening if untreated. Primary concerns include dehydration, hypovolemia, and electrolyte imbalances. The latter can lead to orthostatic hypotension, cardiac arrhythmias, severe fatigue, weakness, and lethargy. With the need for frequent bowel movements and trips to the commode, older adults increase their risk for falls. Rectal pain and excoriation also can occur and increase the risk of infection secondary to open wounds. If patients are bed bound and having difficulty with incontinence, maintaining proper skin integrity is a challenge. Malnutrition, sleep disorders, decreased sexual activity, and fear of eating also may result. Psychological effects, including low self-esteem, depression, and fear of leaving home, can greatly affect the quality of life.

Assessment

The first step in accurately assessing diarrhea is a complete and thorough history and physical examination. Review of the patient's cancer diagnosis, stage, and current treatment is essential. All medication and laxative usage must be reviewed. Obtaining previous bowel history, including an in-depth description of frequency, amount, color, and consistency of stools, is an integral part of assessment. Onset of diarrhea, any associated pain or symptoms, relieving factors, current diet, travel history, and incontinence also should be examined. The physical examination should include weighing the patient, skin turgor assessment, vital signs with lying and standing blood pressures, a comprehensive abdominal exam, rectal exam with occult blood testing, and assessment of the perirectal skin integrity.

Diagnostic and laboratory testing varies according to each individual. However, a basic workup should include a complete blood count, electrolyte panel, and stool analysis for blood (including culture and sensitivity), ova, parasites, white blood cells, and C. *difficile* toxin. In patients with known secretory tumors, urine collection for hydroxyindoleacetic acid or serum vasoactive intestinal protein, gastrin, and calcitonin testing should be considered. Further diagnostic studies, including colonoscopy or barium radiography, eventually may be necessary.

Management

Diarrhea is managed through dietary modification and education about pharmacologic treatments. Prompt management of diarrhea is of great importance to minimize toxicity and associated side effects.

Dietary management should include instruction regarding types of foods to consume as well as interval feeding. The BRAT diet, which includes foods that are bland, low in residue, and rich in potassium (e.g., bananas, rice, apples, toast), is recommended. Milk products, spicy foods, gas-producing vegetables, caffeine, and chocolate should be avoided (Martz, 1996). Smaller, frequent feedings also are recommended. To avoid dehydration, at least three liters of fluid should be consumed per 24 hours (Hogan, 1998). However, caution is necessary in older adults with any history of congestive heart failure or fluid overload. Homecare patients should be encouraged to drink sport drinks or commercial rehydration beverages. In severe cases, hospitalized patients may require total parenteral nutrition.

Pharmacologic treatment of secretory diarrhea consists of the use of opioids, anti-spasmodics, and anticholinergics. Medications used in treating cancer-related diarrhea include loperamide hydrochloride (HCl), atropine sulfate/diphenoxylate HCl, codeine phosphate, octreotide acetate, and bulk-forming and absorbent agents. These medications cause increased transit time, reduced fecal volume, and increased fluid viscosity (Hogan, 1998).

The dose of loperamide HCl is two 2 mg capsules initially, then 2 mg after each loose stool, not to exceed eight capsules per day (Martz, 1996). However, when treating irinotecan-induced diarrhea, the dosage is increased. Possible side effects of loperamide HCl include cramping, gastric upset, and constipation. Loperamide is available over the counter.

Atropine sulfate/diphenoxylate HCl is dosed as one to two tablets three to four times per day, not to exceed eight tablets per day (Martz, 1996). It may cause sedation, dizziness, dry mouth, and urinary retention. The use of this drug is contraindicated in patients with advanced liver disease (Bisanz, 1997). It is also a Schedule V controlled drug requiring prescription.

Codeine sulfate is a Schedule II controlled drug that is much more constipating than morphine and is occasionally used as an antidiarrheal. The recommended dose is 30–60 mg every four to six hours as needed (Bisanz, 1997).

Octreotide acetate is the drug of choice for patients with known endocrine or carcinoid tumors, high-volume diarrhea, and diarrhea resulting from graft-versus-host disease. Octreotide acetate is a synthetic analog of the naturally occurring peptide hormone somatostatin. It acts directly on the epithelial cells of the intestine to inhibit the release of the gastrointestinal hormones, stimulate chloride and sodium absorption, decrease secretion of fluid and electrolytes, and prolong intestinal transit time (Cooper, Williams, King, & Barker, 1986). Octreotide acetate is given as a subcutaneous injection of 50–100 mcg two to three times per day (Martz, 1996). Its side effects include nausea, pain at the injection site, and abdominal cramping.

Other pharmacologic agents used to treat diarrhea include pancreatic enzymes, glutamine, psyllium, bismuth products, and absorbents such as pectin, aluminum, charcoal, and kaolin.

Infections

Patients with fever and bloody or severe diarrhea are likely to be suffering from an infection. With bloody or severe diarrhea, stool cultures should be evaluated and appropriate antibiotic therapy should be started if C. difficile infection is suspected. Oral metronidazole and vancomycin are the antibiotics of choice (Martz, 1996). However, metronidazole is preferred because of its low cost and ease of administration. Patients with C. difficile infection, if hospitalized, must be placed on enteric precautions.

Education

Educating patients and families is a pivotal step in the management of diarrhea. They need to be instructed regarding the potential side effects of treatment, prompt reporting of symptoms, and appropriate prevention and intervention techniques. Nurses have an invaluable role in managing cancer-related diarrhea.

Summary

The management of cancer-related diarrhea in older adults is challenging. It requires a collaborative effort among the patient, the family, and the healthcare team. Early recognition and treatment remains paramount.

Mucositis

Definition and Description

Mucositis is defined as inflammation and/or ulceration of the mucosal membrane (Madeya, 1996a). Mucositis can lead to serious complications, such as septicemia, and can greatly affect quality of life by causing pain and the inability to eat.

Occurrence

The development of oral complications in the cancer population may be a direct result of the disease, the cancer treatment, or other factors affecting oral health. Forty percent of all people newly diagnosed with cancer will develop oral complications, the most common being mucositis (Beck, 1996).

Age-Related Changes

Older adults can be at greater risk for developing mucositis secondary to age-related changes that can occur in the buccal cavity. In older adults, vascularity of the gingiva is reduced, limiting or decreasing the ability of the tissue to heal after injury (Ebersole & Hess, 1998). A loss of submucosal elastin, a loss of connective tissue, and a decrease in the number of minor salivary glands also occur as age increases (Ebersole & Hess). These factors can contribute to increased incidence of mucositis, delayed healing, and increased risk of infection in older adults. Oral cavity assessment methods have improved and awareness concerning mucositis has increased, especially in regard to high-dose chemotherapy and radiation therapy (Berger & Eilers, 1998).

Pathophysiology and Etiology

The oral cavity is composed of a mucosal lining of nonkeritinizing, stratified squamous epithelium. These cells have a high turnover rate and regenerate approximately every 10–14 days (Iwamoto, 1991). This pattern of cellular proliferation makes the mucosa extremely vulnerable to sources of irritation, trauma, and cellular damage, resulting in mucositis. Mucositis can be either disease- or treatment-related. Risk factors for developing mucositis include poor oral hygiene, tobacco and alcohol use, increasing age, impaired nutritional status, dehydration, and oxygen therapy.

Chemotherapy-Induced Mucositis

Mucositis resulting from chemotherapy is caused by a direct effect of the drug on the oral mucosa or an indirect result of the drug's myleosuppressive action (Madeya, 1996a). Only the basal layer of epithelial cells divides and is susceptible to lysis when exposed to chemotherapy or radiation (Rosenberg, 1991). Normally, basal cells divide, and the newly produced cell is displaced upward to the mucosal surface, becoming thin squamous cells that shed. The red, swollen presentation of mucositis results from the exposure of the underlying connective tissue to the oral environment and the tissue's reaction to the insult (Rosenberg).

The direct effect of chemotherapy on the oral mucosa occurs at the cellular level. Chemotherapeutic drugs with the highest stomatotoxic potential include antimetabolites, antitumor antibiotics, plant alkaloids, and taxanes (Beck, 1996) (see Figure 10.7). These drugs cause destruction of mucosal cells that are actively dividing by interfering with DNA, RNA, or protein synthesis. Once the epithelial lining has been disrupted by reduced production, decreased differentiation, or accelerated detachment to the cells, mucositis results from the pattern of tissue destruction, inflammation, and infection. The severity of mucositis varies by drug regimen and dosage, and the intensity of mucositis increases with higher doses of cytotoxic drugs.

Indirect stomatotoxicity is the result of the effects of chemotherapy on the cells of the bone marrow rather than the oral mucosa. Alterations in the oral mucosa correlate with the onset of myelosuppression. Mucositis is observed near the leukocyte nadir and subsequently resolves with the recovery of the marrow (Madeya, 1996a). Indirect stomatotoxicity is believed to be mediated through a suppressed immune response. Patients who are undergoing bone marrow transplant experience severe and prolonged mucositis resulting from the direct stomatotoxic effects of immunosuppressive drugs, total body radiation, and the indirect effects of pancytopenia and aplasia.

Radiation-Induced Mucositis

Mucositis also can result from radiation therapy delivered to the head and neck area. Radiation causes mucosal atrophy because of decreased cell renewal (Madeya, 1996a). An inflammatory response occurs as a result of destruction of the mucosal or glandular cells and is influenced by the depth of penetration, total dose delivered, and number and frequency of treatments. Mucositis usually begins after a dose of about 2,000 cGy and can persist for several weeks after therapy is completed (Beck, 1996). Initially, the mucosa develops erythema and edema, and as treatment continues, the mucosa becomes ulcerated and sloughing occurs. Secondary infections often occur and can prolong the resolution of mucositis.

Clinical Manifestations

The development of mucositis varies from individual to individual. Initially, the oral mucosa may have a slight burning sensation or erythema. This may spontaneously resolve or progress to superficial epithelial desquamation, severe ulceration, pain, glossal edema, and secondary infection (Iwamoto, 1991).

Fungal Complications

Fungi can exist in the oral mucosa when the integrity of the oral mucosa is uninterrupted and protected by rapid cellular renewal (Madeya, 1996a). Disruption of the mucosal barrier can lead to invasive fungal infections. *Candida albicans,* which is part of the normal gastrointestinal and oral flora, is the primary cause of opportunistic fungal disease in immunosuppressed patients. Patients with oral candidiasis are at significant risk of developing esophagitis and systemic candidiasis. Candida usually appears as irregular, white plaques with multiple dome elevations. It involves localized or large areas of the mucosa and usually is preceded by mucositis. It can be diagnosed by

Figure 10.7. Chemotherapy Drugs With High Stomatotoxic Potential

• Fluorouracil	• Vincristine sulfate
• Mitoxantrone	• Doxorubicin
• Methotrexate	• Paclitaxel
• Etoposide	• Mitomycin-C
• Floxuridinex	• Taxotere

fungal cultures and gram stains. Oral candida is treated with nystatin rinses, clotrimazole troches, and oral or IV fluconazole.

Herpetic Complications

Herpetic lesions can be missed easily in a patient with mucositis. These lesions are characterized by single or multiple clusters of small vesicles filled with clear fluid on a raised inflamed base. Oral lesions are most frequently seen on the lips or in the mouth (Madeya, 1996a). In immunocompromised patients, the mucositis associated with herpetic lesions may be more painful and prolonged. The antiviral agent acyclovir is used for the treatment of oral herpes infection.

Hemorrhagic Complications

Hemorrhage from oral mucositis can occur in the presence of thrombocytopenia. The potential for spontaneous bleeding exits when platelet counts fall below 20,000 (Beck & Yasko, 1993). Patients with preexisting periodontal disease or poor oral hygiene are more likely to experience gingival hemorrhage. Local treatment with fibrinolysis inhibitors, such as aminocaproic acid, to bleeding areas can be effective in controlling bleeding; however, platelet transfusion may be necessary. Other complications that can occur secondary to mucositis include pain, taste changes, and xerostomia.

Assessment

Many of the cancer-related oral complications can be avoided, or at least minimized, by a regimen of ongoing assessment. The goals of oral assessment are to maintain tissue integrity and prevent infection. The nurse should obtain the patient's baseline history, including the patient's age, prior oral and dental disease, type of cancer, type of cancer treatment being received, and nutritional status (Madeya, 1996b).

Prior to the exam, the patient should be instructed to remove any dental appliances, especially dentures. An adequate light source also is essential to perform a thorough exam. A tongue blade or dental mirror may facilitate the exam.

Assessment of the oral cavity includes evaluation of the lips, oral mucosa, tongue, saliva, and teeth (Madeya, 1996b). Normal, healthy oral mucosa is intact, pink, and moist. Alterations can include changes in color of the mucosa, including pallor and erythema; open lesions or plaques; changes in moisture; odors; or exudates (Beck, 1996).

The outer and inner lips should be observed, as should the hard and soft palates. The inner cheeks and top and bottom of the tongue also require careful examination. The oropharynx, posterior tongue, and uvula are accessible to direct visualization.

The nurse should take the patient's vital signs to assess temperature and heart rate, which may help to aid in the diagnosis of infection. A complete blood count with differential also is useful, especially in neutropenic and immunocompromised patients. In patients with dysphagia or esophageal pain, endoscopy or swallowing studies may be necessary.

Grading of Mucositis

Mucositis is managed based on the degree of tissue injury. Severity may be graded based on the amount of damage to the mucosa. See Figure 10.8 for grading of mucositis.

Management

Effective management of oral mucositis includes prophylaxis and adequate oral hygiene, as well as symptomatic treatment for pain and infection. Patient and family education also is

Figure 10.8. Grading of Mucositis

Grade 0:	No mucositis; intact oral mucosa without ulceration; pink, soft, and moist
Grade I:	Mild erythema or oral discomfort, with a slight burning sensation
Grade II:	Moderate erythema; shallow ulcerations or white patches; complaints of pain
Grade III:	Confluent ulcerations or white patches covering more than 25% of the oral mucosa, with pain and limited oral intake
Grade IV:	Severe with hemorrhage, ulceration, necrosis, pain, and inability to eat, drink, or swallow

important. Patients who learn to perform regular oral cavity assessment can identify changes earlier and report them more accurately (Madeya, 1996b).

Oral Hygiene

Adequate oral hygiene includes brushing, flossing, rinsing, and moisturizing. Brushing with a soft nylon-bristle toothbrush is effective in removing plaque. Fluoride-containing toothpastes are recommended. Flossing augments the cleaning process by removing debris between teeth. Rinsing with agents such as warm water, salt water, baking soda and water, and half-strength hydrogen peroxide also is recommended (Beck, 1996). Commercial rinses that contain alcohol can irritate and actually dry the mucosa and are not recommended. The lips and mucosa can be kept moist by sucking on sugarless candy or chewing sugarless gum, which stimulate salivary flow. Ointments and lip balms applied to the lips also help.

A large percentage of older adults are edentulous and wear complete dentures. Many elders believe that once they have dentures, there is no longer a need for oral care (Ebersole & Hess). Dentures should be removed at bedtime and replaced in the morning to relieve compression of the gums (Ebersole & Hess, 1998). This also provides an opportunity to view the areas in the mouth normally covered by the dentures. Proper denture care includes soaking in an effervescent cleanser and brushing with a denture brush and paste, followed by thorough rinsing.

Prophylactic interventions aimed at protecting the cells of the mucosa prior to fluorouracil chemotherapy include cryotherapy. Oral cryotherapy consisting of placing ice chips in the mouth before, during, and after chemotherapy causes local vasoconstriction, decreasing oral blood flow (Madeya, 1996b). Mahood et al. (1991) concluded that oral cryotherapy can reduce the incidence of fluorouracil-induced mucositis.

Management of Oral Pain

The most common complication associated with mucositis is pain. Management of oral pain includes the use of anesthetic agents available in sprays, rinses, and gels. These agents are effective within five minutes of application, and the effect lasts for about an hour. They also have very little systemic absorption (Madeya, 1996b). Figure 10.9 lists examples of topical coating agents. These agents form an occlusive film over the oral ulceration and can be used to manage pain from ulcers on the tongue, gums,

Figure 10.9. Topical Coating Agents

- Hurricane® (Beutlich LP Pharmaceuticals, Waukegan, IL)
- Orahesive™ (Convatec Squibb Co., Princeton, NJ)
- Oratect Gel® (MGI Pharmaceuticals Inc., Minneapolis, MN)
- Zilactin™ (Zila Pharmaceuticals, Phoenix, AZ)
- Sucralfate

and mucous membranes inside the cheeks and lips. Commercial topical anesthetic rinses available include dyclonine HCl and MouthKote® (Parnell Pharmaceuticals, Larkspur, CA) oral pain-relief rinse, spray, or gel. These agents contain mucoprotective factor, a natural agent derived from the yerba santa plant, which has moisturizing and lubricating properties (Madeya, 1996b). Combination mixtures of topical anesthetics, anti-inflammatory agents, and antacids also are used to decrease pain and discomfort. An example of one such mixture includes a combination of a 1:1:1 solution of viscous lidocaine, diphenhydramine HCl elixir, and Maalox® (Novartis Consumer Health, Inc.). Patients are instructed to swish and spit or swallow 10 cc of the rinse every four to six hours as needed.

Systematic approaches to the management of mucositis-related pain include the use of analgesics. Lortab® elixir (Whitby Pharmaceuticals, Richmond, VA) has been found to relieve pain associated with radiation-induced esophagitis (Madeya, 1996b). One teaspoon of Lortab contains 12.5 mg hydrocodone barbiturate, 120 mg acetaminophen, and 7% alcohol. Patients are instructed to take one teaspoon one-half hour before meals as needed. The dose may be increased to four teaspoons if necessary (Dunne, 1991).

For moderate mucositis pain, weak opioids are appropriate. Codeine or combinations of hydrocodone and acetaminophen are effective. For unrelieved pain or severe mucositis, strong opioids like oxycodone and morphine may be necessary. Around-the-clock dosing is advantageous, and long-acting preparations of morphine or oxycodone may be beneficial. Continuous IV infusions with patient-controlled analgesia of morphine may eventually be necessary for patient comfort until adequate oral tissue healing has resumed.

Summary

Oral mucositis is a frequent and sometimes severe symptom of cancer and cancer therapy that can greatly affect patients' quality of life. Patient and family education are essential in providing comprehensive care. Routine oral assessment, proper oral hygiene, and aggressive treatment are paramount. Prophylactic behaviors and early intervention can minimize the severity of oral complications. Collaboration among the patient, family, and healthcare team, using a systematic approach, can enhance treatment outcomes.

Conclusion

The symptom management of side effects that occur as the result of cancer and its progression can be modified or ameliorated with accurate assessment and interventions. Planning nursing actions that will provide relief for the patient while reducing the likelihood that the remedies will not compromise the treatments or the patient's quality of life is vitally important to the older adult with cancer. Nursing care of the patient and family are essential throughout the cancer experience.

References

Abbasi, A. (1998). Nutrition. In E. Duthie & P. Katz (Eds.), *Practice of geriatrics* (pp. 145–157). Philadelphia: Saunders.

Agra, Y., Sacristran, A., Gonzalez, M., Portugues, A., & Calvo, M. (1998). Efficacy of senna versus lactulose in terminal cancer patients treated with opioids. *Journal of Pain and Symptom Management, 15,* 1–7.

Ahmedzai, S., & Brooks, D. (1997). Transdermal fentanyl versus sustained relief morphine in cancer pain: Preference, efficacy, and quality of life. *Journal of Pain and Symptom Management, 13,* 254–261.

Allan, S.G. (1992). Antiemetics. *Gastroenterology Clinics of North America, 21,* 597–611.

Beck, S., & Yasko, J. (1993). *Guidelines for oral care* (2nd ed.). Crystal Lake, IL: Sage Products Inc.

Beck, S.L. (1996). Mucositis. In S.L Groenwald, M.H. Frogge, M. Goodman, & C.H. Yarbro (Eds.), *Cancer symptom management* (pp. 308–323). Boston: Jones and Bartlett.

Benton, J.M., O'Hara, P.A., Chen, H., Harper, D.W., & Johnston, S.F. (1997). Changing bowel hygiene practice successfully: A program to reduce laxative use in a chronic care hospital. *Geriatric Nursing, 18*(1), 12–17.

Berger, A.M., & Eilers, J. (1998). Factors influencing oral cavity status during high-dose antineoplastic therapy: A secondary analysis. *Oncology Nursing Forum, 25,* 1623–1626.

Beverly, L., & Travis, I. (1992). Constipation: Proposed natural laxative mixtures. *Journal of Gerontological Nursing, 18*(10), 5–12.

Bisanz, A. (1997). Managing bowel elimination problems in patients with cancer. *Oncology Nursing Forum, 24,* 679–686.

Brocklehurst, J.C. (1992). Constipation and fecal incontinence in old age. In R. Tallis, H. Fillit, & J.C. Brocklehurst (Eds.), *Brocklehurst's textbook of geriatric medicine and gerontology* (5th ed.) (pp. 1329–1341). Edinburgh, Scotland: Churchill Livingstone.

Brown, M.K., & Everett, I. (1990). Gentler bowel fitness with fiber. *Geriatric Nursing, 11*(1), 26–27.

Cameron, J.C. (1992). Constipation related to narcotic therapy. *Cancer Nursing, 15,* 372–377.

Cleri, L.B. (1995). Serotonin antagonists. In S.M. Hubbard, M. Goodman, & T. Knobf (Eds.), *Oncology nursing: Patient treatment and support* (pp. 1 19). Philadelphia: Lippincott.

Cooper, J.C., Williams, N.S., King, R., & Barker, M. (1986). Effects of a long-acting somatostatin analogue in patients with severe ileostomy diarrhea. *British Journal of Surgery, 73,* 128–131.

Culpepper-Morgan, J.A., Inturrisi, C.E., Portenoy, R.K., Foley, K., Houde, R.W., Marsh, F., & Kreek, M.J. (1992). Treatment of opioid-induced constipation with oral naloxone: A pilot study. *Clinical Trials and Therapeutics, 52,* 90–95.

Dodd, M., Onishki, K., Dibble, S., & Larson, P. (1996). Differences in nausea, vomiting, and retching between younger and older outpatients receiving cancer chemotherapy. *Cancer Nursing, 19,* 155–161.

Dunne, C. (1991). Oral analgesics to relieve radiation-induced esophagitis. *Oncology Nursing Forum, 18,* 785.

Ebersole, P., & Hess, P. (1998). *Toward healthy aging: Human needs and nursing response* (5th ed.). St. Louis: Mosby.

Engelking, C. (1998). Cancer treatment-related diarrhea: Challenges and barriers to clinical practice. In S.M. Hubbard, M. Goodman, & M.T. Knobf (Eds.), *Oncology nursing updates, patient treatment, and support* (pp. 1–12). Cedar Knolls, NJ: Lippincott Williams & Wilkins.

Gross, J. (1994). Functional alterations: Bowel. In J. Gross & B.L. Johnston (Eds.), *Handbook of oncology nursing* (2nd ed.) (pp. 517–528). Boston: Jones and Bartlett.

Hogan, C.M. (1998). The nurse's role in diarrhea management. *Oncology Nursing Forum, 25,* 879–886.

Ippoliti, C., & Neumann, J. (1998). Octreotide in the management of diarrhea induced by graft versus host disease. *Oncology Nursing Forum, 25,* 873–878.

Iwamoto, R.R. (1991). Alterations in oral status. In S.B. Baird, R. McCorkle, & M. Grant (Eds.), *Cancer nursing: A comprehensive textbook* (pp. 742–758). Philadelphia: Saunders.

Jenns, K. (1994). Importance of nausea. *Cancer Nursing, 17,* 488–493.

Kris, M.G., Tyson, L.B., Gralla, R.J., Clark, R.A., Allen, J.C., & Reilly, L.K. (1983). Extra-pyramidal reactions with high dose metoclopramide [Letter to the editor]. *New England Journal of Medicine, 309,* 433.

Latreille, J., Pater, J., Johnston, D., LaBerge, F., Stewart, D., Rusthoven, J., Hoskins, P., Findlay, B., McMurtrie, E., Yelle, L., Williams, C., Walde, D., Ernst, S., Dhaliwal, H., Warr, D., Shepherd, F., Mee, D., Nishimura, L., Osoba, D., & Zee, B. (1998). Use of dexamethasone and granisetron in the control of delayed emesis for patients who receive highly emetogenic chemotherapy. *Journal of Clinical Oncology, 16,* 1174–1178.

Levy, M.H. (1992). Constipation and diarrhea in cancer patients. *Cancer Bulletin, 43,* 412–422.

Madeya, M.L. (1996a). Oral complications from cancer therapy: Part 1—Pathophysiology and secondary complications. *Oncology Nursing Forum, 23,* 801–807.

Madeya, M.L. (1996b). Oral complications from cancer therapy: Part 2—Nursing implications for assessment and treatment. *Oncology Nursing Forum, 23,* 808–819.

Mahood, D., Dose, A., Loprinzi, C., Veeder, M., Anthman, L., Therneau, T.M., Sorensen, J., Gainey, D., Mailliard, J., Gusa, N., Fink, G., Johnson, C., & Goldberg, R. (1991). Inhibition of fluorouracil-induced stomatitis by oral cryotherapy. *Journal of Clinical Oncology, 9,* 449–452.

Martz, C.H. (1996). Diarrhea. In S.L. Groenwald, M.H. Frogge, M. Goodman, & C.H. Yarbro (Eds.), *Cancer symptom management* (pp. 498–520). Boston: Jones and Bartlett.

Mercandante, S. (1995). Diarrhea in terminally ill patients: Pathophysiology and treatment. *Journal of Pain and Symptom Management, 10,* 298–308.

Mercandante, S. (1998). Diarrhea, malabsorption, and constipation. In A.M. Berger, R.K. Portenoy, & D.E. Weissman (Eds.), *Principles and practice of supportive oncology* (pp. 191–205). Philadelphia: Lippincott-Raven.

Mystakidou, K., Befon, S., Liossi, C., & Vlachos, L. (1998). Comparison of tropisetron and chlorpromazine in the control of nausea and vomiting in patients with advanced cancer. *Journal of Pain and Symptom Management, 15,* 176–184.

Pisters, K.M.W., & Kris, M.G. (1998). Treatment-related nausea and vomiting. In A.W. Berger, M.R.K. Portenoy, & D.E. Weissman (Eds.), *Principles and practice of supportive oncology* (pp. 165–177). Philadelphia: Lippincott-Raven.

Portenoy, R.K. (1987). Constipation in the cancer patient. *Medical Clinics of North America, 71,* 303–311.

Reuben, D.B., & Mor, V. (1986). Nausea and vomiting in terminal cancer patients. *Archives of Internal Medicine, 146,* 2021–2023.

Rosenberg, S.W. (1991). The Sonis/Clark article reviewed. Prevention and management of oral mucositis induced by antineoplastic therapy. *Oncology, 12,* 18.

Rutledge, D.N., & Engelking, C. (1998). Cancer-related diarrhea: Selected findings of a national survey of oncology nurse experiences. *Oncology Nursing Forum, 25,* 861–872.

Schuster, M. (1994). Gastroparesis. In T.M. Bayless (Ed.), *Current therapy in gastroenterology and liver disease* (pp. 151–154). St. Louis: Mosby.

Sykes, N.P. (1996). An investigation of the ability of oral naloxone to correct opioid-related constipation in patients with advanced cancer. *Palliative Medicine, 10,* 135–144.

Wadler, S., Benson, A.B., Engelking, C., Catalano, R., Field, M., Kornblau, S.M., Mitchell, E., Rubin, J., Trotta, P., & Vokes, E. (1998). Recommended guidelines for the treatment of chemotherapy-induced diarrhea. *Journal of Clinical Oncology, 16,* 3169–3178.

Wickham, R. (1996). Nausea and vomiting. In S.L. Groenwald, M.H. Frogge, M. Goodman, & C.H. Yarbro (Eds.), *Cancer symptom management* (pp. 218–251). Boston: Jones and Bartlett.

Violette, K.M. (1998). Nausea and vomiting. In C.R. Ziegfeld, B.G. Lubejejko, & B.K. Shelton (Eds.), *Manual of cancer care* (pp. 335–344). Philadelphia: Lippincott.

Yakabowich, M. (1990). Prescribe with care: The role of laxatives in the treatment of constipation. *Journal of Gerontological Nursing, 16*(7), 4–11.

Chapter Eleven

Quality-of-Life Assessment for the Older Adult With Cancer

Enoch Albert, MS, RNC, OCN®

Rationale for Assessing Quality of Life

The quality-of-life (QOL) assessment is widely accepted as part of the total assessment of patient outcomes during clinical trials of new cancer treatments. It has been extensively studied in recent years within the research community (Bennahum, Forman, Vellas, & Albarede, 1997; Bland, 1997; Cella & Bonomi, 1995; Gralla & Moinpour, 1995; King et al., 1997; Post-White et al., 1996; Turner, 1997). Cella and Bonomi noted that the U.S. Food and Drug Administration (FDA) regards the benefits to patient QOL as one of the major requirements for approval of new anticancer drugs.

A growing consensus within the healthcare community indicates that the therapeutic effectiveness of clinical trials must be assessed with regard to the quality as well as the quantity of patient survival (King et al., 1997). Balancing cure and care is an important concept in the treatment of people of all ages who have cancer, but it is especially relevant for older adults with cancer (Bennahum et al., 1997). Bennahum et al. identified the importance of physicians and nurses recognizing that QOL can be measured and should be part of every treatment plan. Although QOL assessment is well accepted and used in clinical trials, it is not commonly used as a general clinical practice tool.

QOL in Clinical Practice

Several reasons for assessing QOL include
- Screening patients on a scheduled basis for previously identified and new problems
- Monitoring patients' progress and response to therapy
- Helping patients and physicians make decisions about alternative treatment regimens (Bennahum et al., 1997).

When patients experience a decline in QOL, consideration should be given to decreasing the intensity of cancer therapy.

Providers

Providers need to discuss the personal meaning of QOL with elderly patients to determine the treatment preferences of each individual. Some elderly patients are concerned with living longer and improving, or at least maintaining, their current state of living. Some older adults with cancer want to have clear cognition and freedom from pain. Other patients will trade one aspect of QOL for another if given sufficient information concerning the choices.

Individualizing the care plan to meet the unique needs of older adults with cancer should be a goal of nursing care. During the initial interview, specific information related to the person's preferences for QOL should be obtained. With some patients, this assessment can be obtained very easily; for others, it may be more challenging or incomplete because of a number of factors. For instance, some older adults may be reluctant to discuss personal matters. Some patients have sensory or memory limitations or mental status changes. A standardized assessment tool can help to ensure consistent results across patients and practitioners. When an assessment tool is effective, it can stimulate patients to remember problems that they may not have discussed otherwise. The author has noted that American men may be reluctant to discuss personal matters with healthcare providers who are unknown to them. This less-than-trusting attitude can adversely affect the plan of treatment.

Capra (1996) noted that much of scientific thinking is concentrated on the "study of substance," which traces its roots to the Greek philosophers of the sixth century B.C. This direction in scientific thinking has produced an incredible body of knowledge about living systems, including the basis of modern medical practice. However, Capra recognized a "tension" between this study of substance and the study of form or patterns, which also had its beginning in ancient Greece. Today, this latter study is known as systems theory. Capra proposed a synthesis of these two approaches as the key to understanding living systems. The holistic approach to health care, which can be enhanced by assessing and addressing QOL issues of patients, embodies such a synthesis.

Using a QOL instrument to look at the physical, psychosocial, and spiritual aspects of a person provides a basic understanding of the pattern of older adults with cancer, which is necessary to help the older adult with cancer to cope with the disease. One approach to obtaining information from the patient is a mechanistic method (i.e., looking at the substance, according to Capra's terminology). This method enables the nurse to focus energy on issues that are important at a specific point in the patient's life then to prioritize care toward the patient's identified problems.

Selecting an Appropriate QOL Tool

Cella and Bonomi (1995) discussed the difficulty of choosing an assessment instrument for measuring QOL and noted four required attributes of an assessment tool. The tool should
1. Demonstrate a clear and significant contribution to patient care.
2. Not constitute an unacceptable burden to patients or staff.
3. Be sufficiently sensitive to meet the needs of the investigator.
4. Be perceived as unintrusive to patients and the treating staff.
Cella and Bonomi noted that no "gold standard" exists for QOL assessment (i.e., no one best tool to choose or to use to compare with other tools). In addition, no single accepted definition

of QOL currently exists, and some researchers contend that establishing one definition may not be possible (King et al., 1997). Thus, it is up to individual healthcare providers to determine what information is necessary and then select the tool that will elicit the information for that specific issue (e.g., nutrition, pain).

For clinical nursing practice, selecting an assessment tool is further complicated because most QOL tools have been developed for research purposes. They tend to be very long and detailed, therefore requiring a significant expenditure of time and energy to administer. Siu et al. (1993) tested the validity of using several different QOL tools with older adults and concluded that short measures, such as the Dartmouth COOP Project Functional Assessment Charts (Trustees of Dartmouth College, 1996), can be used for elderly individuals, even those with mildly impaired cognitive function.

Schag and Heinrich's Cancer Rehabilitation Evaluation System (CARES) instrument, which has a short form for clinical use and a long form for research purposes, also has been recommended (King et al., 1997). Cella and Bonomi (1995) recognized the short form, which contains 59 items, as best used in research settings. They also concluded that it was not designed with older adults in mind.

Eliopoulos (1995) suggested that the Katz Index of Activities of Daily Living (ADL) be used with older adults. However, this tool does not deal with issues common to patients with cancer, such as pain and nausea and vomiting. The Katz Index of ADLs requires that a trained person be available to determine the patient's score. This can place an undue burden on healthcare facilities when other scales are available that can be scored by nurse clinicians.

No commonly recognized tool for assessing QOL in older adults appears to be available. This does not, however, lead to the conclusion that nurses should not attempt to make QOL assessments of older adults with cancer. Given the quantity of QOL instruments, some researchers have wisely recommended that new instruments should only be developed when existing ones cannot be adapted to a given population (King et al., 1997).

Using Dartmouth COOP Charts

The COOP Charts are designed to screen or monitor function and health-related QOL issues (Nelson et al., 1987). This system consists of nine charts that can be administered by nurses or other designated support staff, or they may be self-administered. Three additional charts have been developed by this author to provide additional information that is important to older adults with cancer. The COOP Charts and additional charts are shown in Figures 11.1 through 11.12.

To use the COOP Charts, the patient reads a chart and then selects the one answer that best reflects his or her status. The entire process can be completed in about five minutes when self-administered; thus, the charts are well-suited to a busy clinical practice or unit. If the nurse clinician desires to keep a record for each patient, the scores can be quickly recorded in the patient record or on a separate data sheet. The graphic figures on the charts enhance their usefulness for older patients with limited literacy (eighth-grade reading level or less) or limited English skills. In addition, the COOP Charts are available in Spanish, Japanese, Hebrew, Dutch, German, and Finnish.

The COOP Charts have been tested for validity and reliability on more than 2,000 patients in four diverse clinical settings and were found to be both valid and reliable (Nelson, Landgraf, Hayes, Wasson, & Kirk, 1990). The charts were used to test the validity of using brief measures of health and self-reported physical functioning of 155 very old people (mean age of 84.3 years). Both convergent and discriminant validity were found to be similar to that observed in studies of the nonelderly (Siu et al., 1993).

Figure 11.1. COOP Chart: Physical Fitness

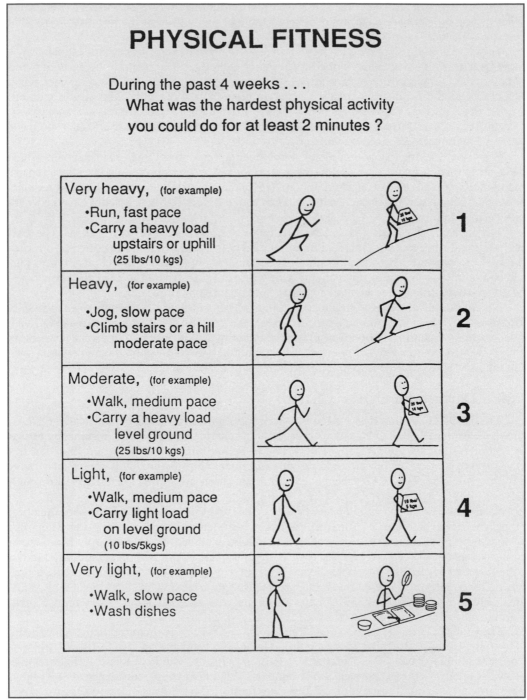

Figure 11.2. COOP Chart: Feelings

FEELINGS

During the past 4 weeks . . .
How much have you been bothered by
emotional problems such as feeling anxious,
depressed, irritable or downhearted and blue ?

Not at all	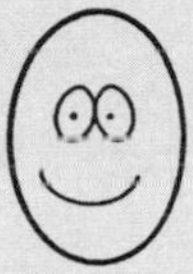 🙂	**1**
Slightly	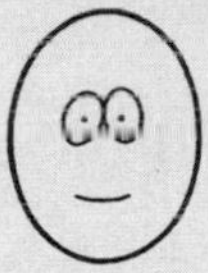 🙂	**2**
Moderately	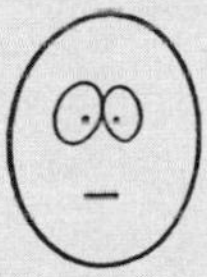 😐	**3**
Quite a bit	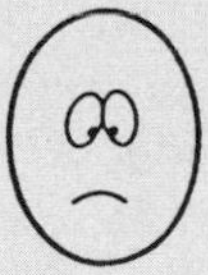 🙁	**4**
Extremely	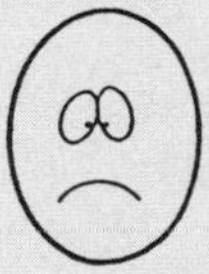 🙁	**5**

Note. Copyright Trustees of Dartmouth College/COOP Project, 1996. Reprinted with permission.

Figure 11.3. COOP Chart: Daily Activities

DAILY ACTIVITIES

During the past 4 weeks . . .
How much difficulty have you had doing your usual
activities or task, both inside and outside the house
because of your physical and emotional health ?

No difficulty at all	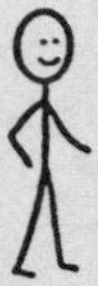	1
A little bit of difficulty	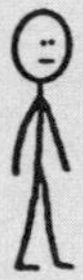	2
Some difficulty	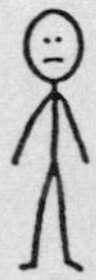	3
Much difficulty	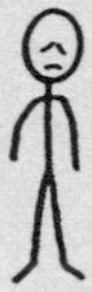	4
Could not do	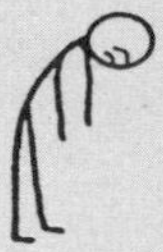	5

Note. Copyright Trustees of Dartmouth College/COOP Project, 1996. Reprinted with permission.

Figure 11.4. COOP Chart: Pain

PAIN

During the past 4 weeks . . .
How much bodily pain have you
generally had ?

No pain	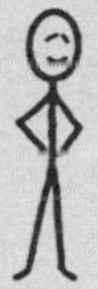	1
Very mild pain	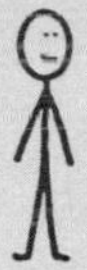	2
Mild pain	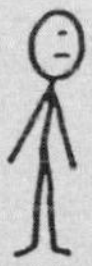	3
Moderate pain	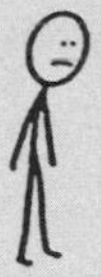	4
Severe pain	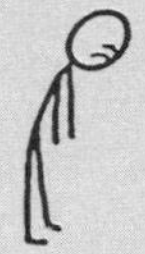	5

Figure 11.5. COOP Chart: Overall Health

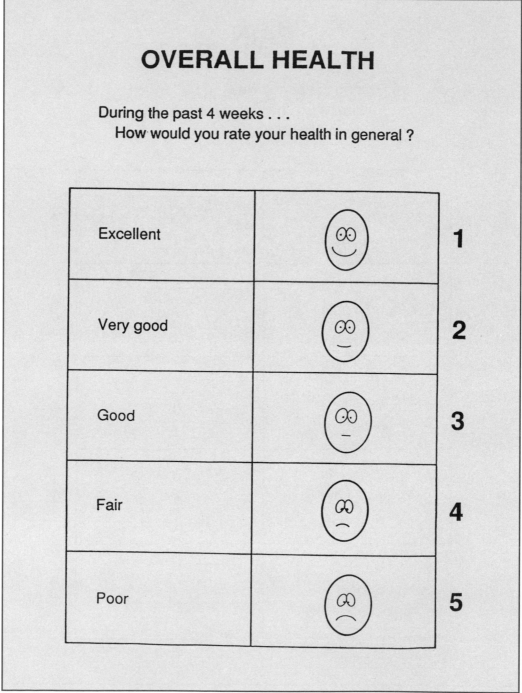

Figure 11.6. COOP Charts: Social Support

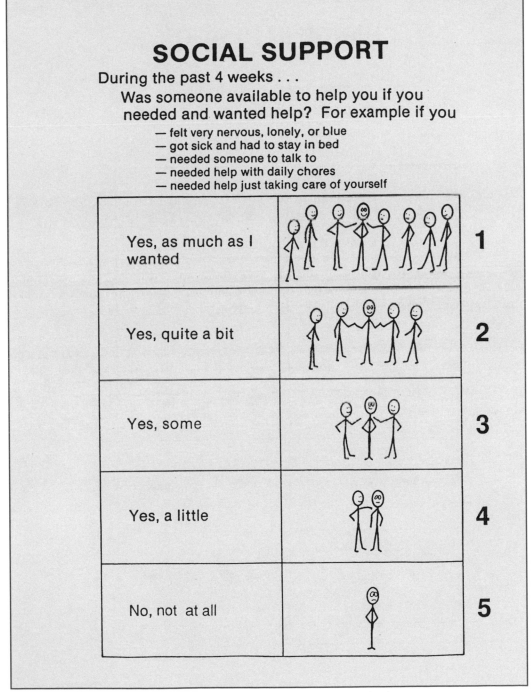

SOCIAL SUPPORT

During the past 4 weeks . . .

Was someone available to help you if you needed and wanted help? For example if you

— felt very nervous, lonely, or blue
— got sick and had to stay in bed
— needed someone to talk to
— needed help with daily chores
— needed help just taking care of yourself

Yes, as much as I wanted		1
Yes, quite a bit		2
Yes, some		3
Yes, a little		4
No, not at all		5

Note. Copyright Trustees of Dartmouth College/COOP Project, 1996. Reprinted with permission.

Figures 11.7. COOP Chart: Change in Health

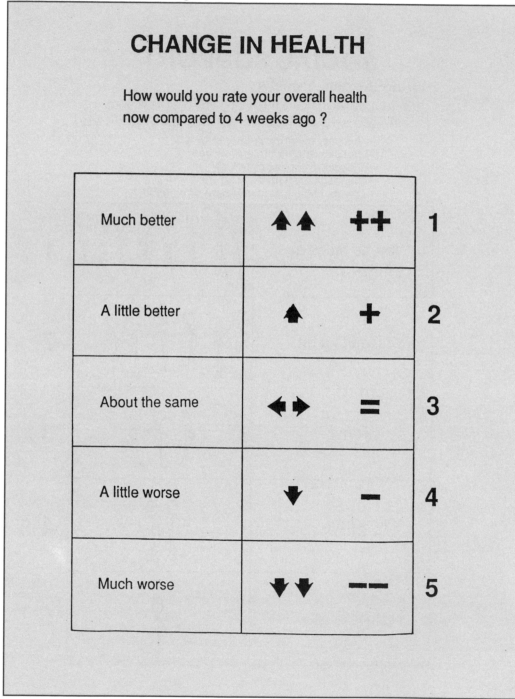

Figures 11.8. COOP Chart: Social Activities

SOCIAL ACTIVITIES

During the past 4 weeks . . .
   Has your physical and emotional health limited
   your social activities with family, friends,
   neighbors or groups ?

Not at all	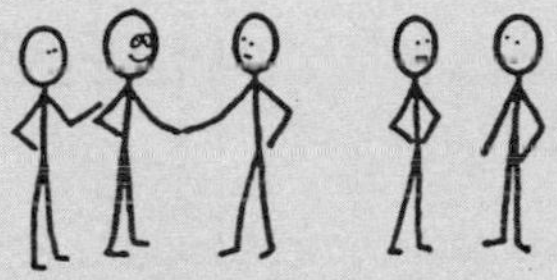	1
Slightly	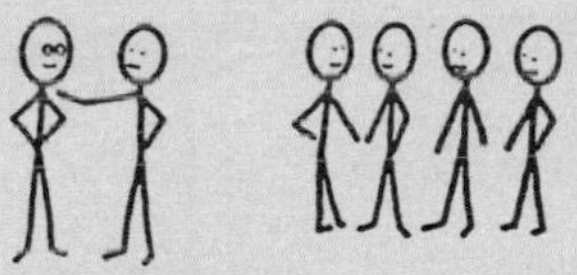	2
Moderately	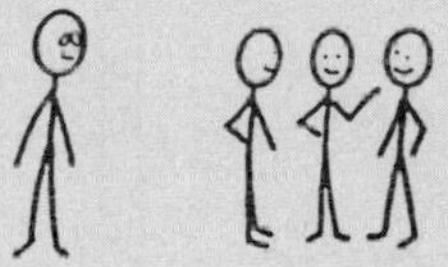	3
Quite a bit	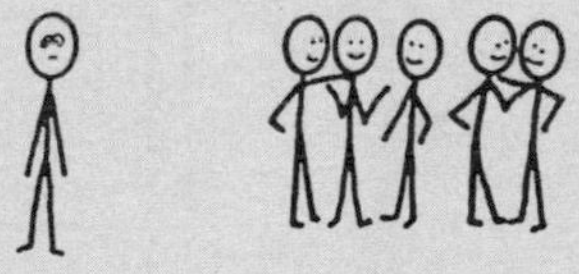	4
Extremely	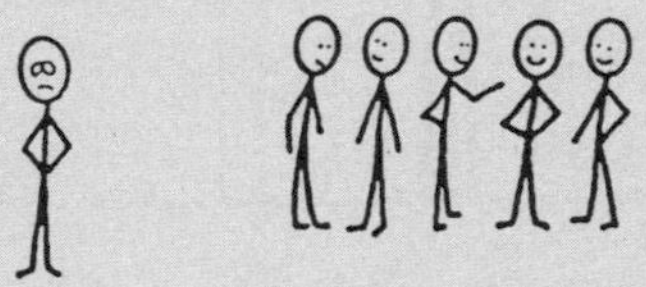	5

Figure 11.9. COOP Chart: Quality of Life

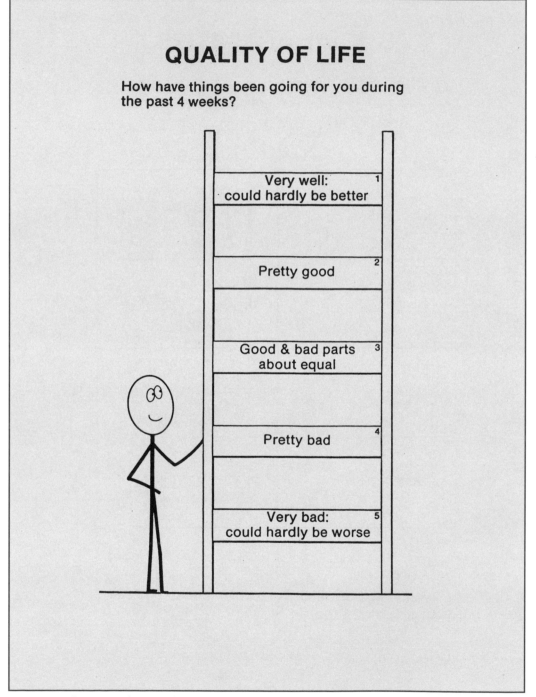

Figure 11.10. Marriage/Sexuality Issues Chart

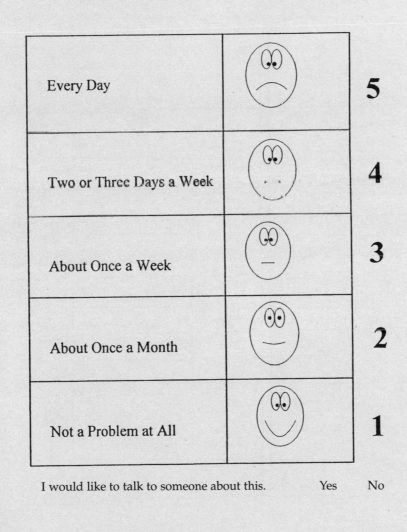

MARRIAGE/SEXUALITY ISSUES

Do you have concerns or problems about your marriage or sexuality that bother you or your spouse?   This happens:

Every Day		5
Two or Three Days a Week		4
About Once a Week		3
About Once a Month		2
Not a Problem at All		1

I would like to talk to someone about this.   Yes   No

Note. Printed with permission from Enoch Albert, copyright 1999.

Figure 11.11. Spiritual/Religious Needs Chart

SPIRITUAL/RELIGIOUS NEEDS

I feel the need to talk or pray with someone about spiritual issues because my needs are not being met. This happens:

Every Day	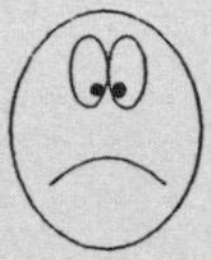	5
Two or Three Days a Week	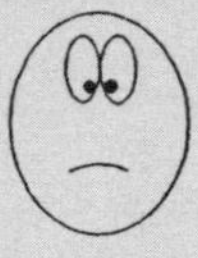	4
About Once a Week	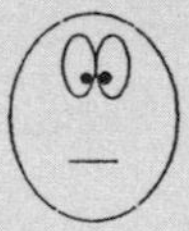	3
About Once a Month	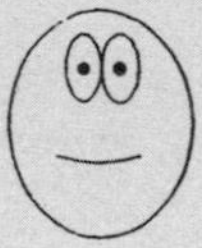	2
Not at All	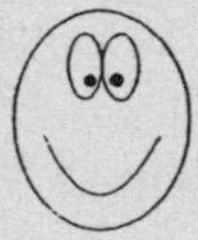	1

I would like to talk to someone about this.   Yes   No

Note. Printed with permission from Enoch Albert, copyright 1999.

Figure 11.12. Food Issues Chart

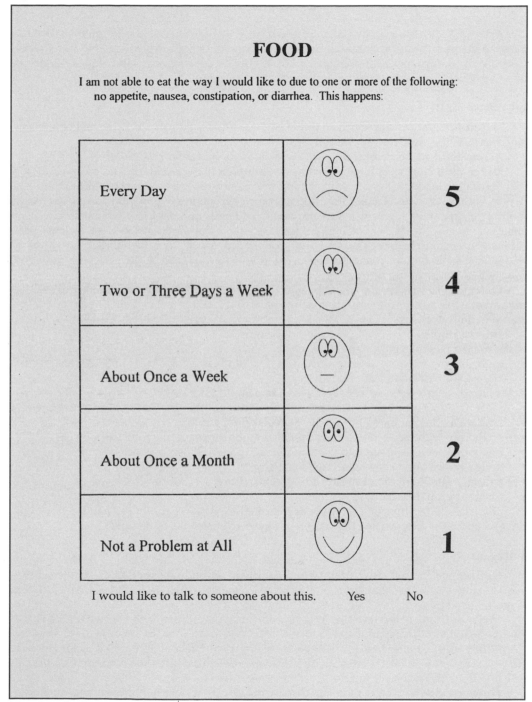

Note. Printed with permission from Enoch Albert, copyright 1999.

Nursing Interventions

After QOL is assessed, the patient's needs must be identified and nursing interventions must be planned. Using the nursing process with nursing diagnoses will enable the clinician to establish an appropriate nursing care plan. The following diagnoses and nursing interventions have been found to benefit elderly patients with cancer (Carpenito, 1997).

Chronic Pain

Definition: The state in which an individual experiences pain that is persistent or intermittent and lasts for more than six months

Major defining characteristic: Pain has existed for more than six months

Older adult considerations: Pain may be omnipresent in the elderly and accepted as normal, leading to inadequate pain management. The elderly may not demonstrate objective signs of pain because of years of adaptation and tolerance; acceptance of pain may lead to decreased mobility; pain-coping mechanisms are important to identify and reinforce in pain management; effects of narcotics are prolonged in the elderly because of decreased metabolism and clearance; side effects seem to be more frequent and pronounced, especially anticholinergic, extrapyramidal, and sedation; drugs should be started at lower doses than in the general population; drug interactions should be monitored.

Outcome criteria: The person will relate that pain is validated by others; practice selected noninvasive pain-relief measures to manage pain; and relate improvement of pain and an increase in daily activities.

Interventions:
- Assess the patient's pain experience.
- Determine the intensity of the pain at its worst and best using a quantifiable scale.
- Assess for factors that decrease pain tolerance.
- Reduce or eliminate factors that increase the pain experience.
- Assess effects of chronic pain on the patient's life, including assessment of both patient and family.
- Assist the patient and family to reduce effects of depression.
- Collaborate with the patient to determine methods to reduce the intensity of pain.
- Collaborate with the patient to use noninvasive pain-relief measures.
- Provide information about prescribed analgesics.
- Reduce or eliminate common side effects of narcotics.
- Promote optimal mobility.
- Initiate health teaching and referrals as indicated.

See Chapter 9 for an extensive discussion of cancer pain and the older adult.

Fatigue

Definition: The self-recognized state in which an individual experiences an overwhelming, sustained sense of exhaustion and decreased capacity for physical and mental work that is not relieved by rest

Major defining characteristics: Verbalization of an unremitting and overwhelming lack of energy; inability to maintain usual routines

Older adult considerations: Fatigue is not a normal effect of aging; risk factors include chronic diseases, medications, treatment, and anemia; late-life depression is common in the elderly and does cause chronic fatigue.

Outcome criteria: The person will discuss the causes of fatigue; share feelings regarding the effects of fatigue on daily life; establish priorities for daily and weekly activities; and participate in activities that stimulate and balance physical, cognitive, affective, and social domains.

Interventions:

- Assess causative or contributing factors.
- Explain the causes of fatigue.
- Allow expression of feelings regarding the effects of fatigue on life.
- Assist the individual to identify strengths, abilities, and interests.
- Assist the individual to identify energy patterns and the need to schedule activities.
- Assist the individual to identify what tasks can be delegated.
- Explain the purpose of pacing and prioritization.
- Teach energy-conservation techniques.
- Explain the effects of conflict and stress on energy levels, and assist the patient in learning effective coping skills.
- Explain the psychological and physiologic benefits of exercise, and discuss what is realistic.
- Provide significant others with an opportunity to discuss feelings in private.
- Initiate health teaching and referrals as needed.

Altered Nutrition: Less Than Body Requirements

Definition: The state in which an individual who is capable of eating experiences or is at risk of having reduced weight related to inadequate intake or poor metabolism of nutrients for metabolic needs

Major defining characteristics: Inadequate food intake less than the recommended daily allowance (RDA) with or without weight loss and/or actual or potential metabolic needs in excess of intake with associated weight loss

Older adult considerations: Elderly adults need the same balanced diet as younger adults, with the exception of fewer calories; individuals who are taking diuretics should be assessed for adequate fluid and electrolyte balance; assess for anemia.

Outcome criteria: Daily nutritional requirements will be met in accordance with activity level and metabolic needs.

Interventions:

- Explain the need for adequate consumption of carbohydrates, fats, protein, vitamins, minerals, and fluids.
- Consult with a nutritionist to establish appropriate daily caloric and food type requirements.
- Discuss possible causes of decreased appetite.
- Encourage rest before meals.
- Suggest small, frequent meals.
- Serve cold foods.
- Restrict liquids with meals and one hour before and after meals.
- Encourage or provide good oral hygiene.
- Take steps to promote appetite (e.g., identify food preferences, promote a relaxed atmosphere and socialization during meals).
- Provide written guidelines on nutrition (e.g., increase complex carbohydrates and fiber; decrease sugar, salt, cholesterol, total fat, and saturated fats; moderate alcohol consumption).
- Assess for factors that interfere with nutrition (e.g., anorexia caused by medications, grief, depression, illness, impaired mental status, impaired mobility, fear of urinary incontinence, history of malnutrition, poor dentition or new dentures, lack of transportation to store, inability to cook).

- Consult with home health nurse to evaluate home environment.
- Access community agencies (e.g., Meals on Wheels, USDA Food Stamp Program).

Constipation Related to Narcotic Administration or Chemotherapy

Definition: The state in which a patient experiences or is at high risk of experiencing stasis of the large intestine resulting in infrequent elimination and/or hard, dry feces

Major defining characteristics: Hard, formed stool and/or defecation occurring fewer than three times a week

Older adult considerations: Current research has not validated that older adults are at higher risk for constipation because of age-related changes; some are prone to constipation because of decreased activity, insufficient dietary fiber and bulk, insufficient fluid intake, side effects of medications, laxative abuse, and inattention to defecation cues.

Outcome criteria: The patient will initiate a therapeutic bowel regimen, relate or demonstrate improved bowel elimination, explain rationale for interventions.

Interventions:
- Assess contributing factors, including side effects of medical regimen, inadequate exercise, imbalanced diet, irregular schedule, and stress.
- Promote corrective measures, including regular time for elimination.
- Identify normal defecation pattern before constipation develops.
- Provide stimulus to defecation, such as coffee or prune juice.
- Advise patient to attempt to defecate about an hour after meals.
- Encourage use of bathroom instead of bedpan, if possible.
- Provide for privacy by closing door, drawing curtains around bed, playing television or radio to mask sounds, and having room deodorizer available.
- Provide for comfort with reading material as a diversion and for safety with a call bell available.
- Provide for moderate physical exercise on a frequent basis if not contraindicated.
- Teach exercises for increased abdominal muscle tone unless contraindicated, including contracting abdominal muscles several times frequently throughout the day, doing sit-ups, keeping heels on floor with knees slightly flexed, and lying supine and raising lower limbs while keeping knees straight.
- Review list of foods with high bulk, including fresh fruits with skins, bran, nuts and seeds, whole-grain breads and cereals, cooked fruits and vegetables, and fruit juices.
- Discuss dietary preferences, taking into account any food intolerances or allergies.
- Encourage consumption of four servings of fresh fruit and a large salad to promote normal daily bowel movement; suggest use of bran in moderation initially because it may irritate the gastrointestinal tract, produce flatulence, and cause diarrhea or blockage; gradually increase amount of bran as tolerated.
- Encourage intake of at least 8–10 glasses of fluids unless contraindicated; recommend a glass of hot water taken one-half hour before breakfast, which may act as a stimulus to bowel evacuation.
- Assist patient to assume a normal semi-squatting position to allow optimal use of abdominal muscles and effects of gravity.
- Stress avoidance of straining, and encourage exhaling during defecation.
- Place a call bell within easy reach.
- Chart color, consistency, and amount of stool.
- Assess elimination status when patient is receiving certain narcotic analgesics, and alert primary healthcare provider if patient is experiencing difficulty with defecation.

- Conduct health teaching for patient and family, explain the relationship of lifestyle changes or medications to constipation, and explain interventions that relieve symptoms and techniques to reduce the effects of stress and immobility.

Ineffective Coping Related to Cancer Survivorship Issues, Cancer Recurrence, or Terminal Diagnosis

Definition: Patient experiences, or is at risk to experience, an inability to adequately manage internal or environmental stressors because of inadequate resources (physical, psychological, behavioral, and/or cognitive); a patient may respond to overwhelming stress with a grief response, such as denial, anger, or sadness, making "grieving" the appropriate nursing diagnosis

Major defining characteristics: Verbalization of inability to cope or ask for help, inappropriate use of defense mechanisms, or inability to meet role expectations

Older adult considerations: Chronic illness has been identified as one of the major psychosocial challenges of older adults; coping is facilitated in those with higher incomes, higher occupational status, and feelings of high self-efficacy (however, when significant life changes are necessary, higher occupational status and feelings of high self-efficacy may be liabilities because these individuals may hold an unrealistic view of what is controllable); a number of events in a short period of time represents the greatest challenge to older adults.

Outcome criteria: The patient will verbalize feelings related to emotional state; identify coping patterns and consequences of resulting behavior; identify personal strengths and accept support through nursing relationships; and make decisions and follow through with appropriate actions.

Interventions:
- Assess for risk factors (e.g., inadequate economic resources, immature developmental level, unanticipated stressful events, occurrence of several major events in a short period of time, unrealistic goals).
- Assess causative and contributing factors (e.g., inadequate problem solving, loss-related grief, sudden change in life pattern, inadequate support system, recent change in health status of patient or significant other).
- Establish rapport; spend time with individual and allow extra time for person to respond; convey honesty and empathy; avoid being overly cheerful; avoid clichés such as "Things will be better"; and do not argue with expressions of worthlessness by saying things such as "How can you say that? Look at all you accomplished in life."
- Encourage expression of feelings and offer support.
- Determine risk of self-harm and intervene appropriately.
- Assess level of depression and intervene according to level; severely depressed or suicidal individuals need environmental controls, usually hospitalization; severely depressed people need assistance with decision making, grooming, hygiene, and nutrition; involve them in activities; do not allow social withdrawal.
- Mobilize into a gradual increase in activities, especially those that previously were gratifying but have been neglected; find outlets that foster feelings of personal achievement and self-esteem.
- Facilitate emotional support from others.
- Initiate health teaching and referrals for depression-related problems beyond the scope of nurse generalist; refer to marriage counselor, psychiatric nurse therapist, psychologist, or psychiatrist as needed.
- Instruct the individual in relaxation techniques; emphasize the importance of setting 15–20 minutes aside each day to practice relaxation or meditation.

Grieving Related to Loss of Function or Independence, Surgery, Chronic Pain, or Terminal Illness

Definition: A state in which the patient or family experience a natural human response involving psychosocial and physiologic reactions to an actual or perceived loss (e.g., person, object, function, status, relationship)

Major defining characteristic: Reporting of an actual or perceived loss

Older adult considerations: Grief may be related to decreased body function and may be less easily accepted than the loss of a significant other; about 25% of all suicides are committed by older adults; reminiscence therapy or life review can help to integrate losses; social supports, strong religious beliefs, good prior mental health, and a greater number of resources are related to less psychosocial or physical dysfunction.

Outcome criteria: The patient will provide personal expressions of grief and be able to describe the meaning of the loss and be able to share grief with significant others (e.g., children, spouses).

Interventions:

- Assess for causative and contributing factors that may delay the grief work (e.g., unavailability or lack of support system, multiple losses, history of previous emotional illness, personality structure).
- Reduce or eliminate causative or contributing factors, if possible, by promoting a trusting relationship.
- Support the patient's and the family's grief reactions.
- Promote family cohesiveness.
- Promote grief work: Recognize that denial is a useful and necessary response, explain the use of denial by one family member to the other members, do not push patient to move past denial without emotional readiness, and create open, honest communications to promote sharing.
- Inform the patient and family that they may experience avoidance from some friends and family who may not be comfortable with their situation of loss or their grief responses.
- Encourage the patient and family to let significant others know what their needs are.
- Identify the level of depression, and develop the approach accordingly.
- Identify any indications of suicidal behavior.
- Understand that anger usually replaces denial; explain to the family that anger is an attempt to try to control one's environment more closely because of inability to control loss.
- Stress that the illness did not result from being a bad person.
- Promote physical well-being (e.g., nutrition, rest, exercise).
- Provide health teaching and referrals.
- Teach the patient and family signs of resolution (e.g., patient is future-oriented and establishes new goals, patient begins to resocialize).
- Identify agencies that may be helpful (e.g., community agencies, religious groups).

Altered Sexuality Patterns Related to Disease Process or Treatment

Definition: The state in which a patient experiences or is at risk of experiencing a change in sexual behaviors or sexual health

Major defining characteristics: Actual or anticipated negative changes in sexual behaviors, sexual health, sexual functioning, or sexual identity

Older adult considerations: Older adults are psychologically and physically capable of engaging in sexual activity regardless of changes in sexual anatomy and physiology caused by aging; sexual activity often is beneficial for the older adult, reducing anxiety while providing intimacy and improving QOL; women experience decreased breast tone, thinning and loss of elasticity of the vaginal wall, deceased vaginal lubrication, and shortening of vaginal length caused by the loss of circulating estrogen; men experience decreased production of spermatozoa, decreased ejaculatory force, and smaller and less firm testicles; direct stimulation may be required to achieve an erection, but the erection may be maintained for a longer time; the need for intimacy and touch is especially important for the older adult who may be experiencing diminishing meaningful relationships; past sexual function is a predictor of sexual activity, and to be capable of sexual activity in old age, the patient will have participated in sexual activity throughout life; adult children and caregivers commonly view sexual activities of older adults as immoral, inappropriate, or negative; the sexual functioning of older adults often is influenced by myths and misunderstanding.

Outcome criteria: The patient will identify the impact of stressors and the loss or change of sexual functioning; modify behavior to reduce stressors; resume previous sexual activity, or engage in alternate satisfying sexual activity; identify factual limitations on sexual activity caused by health problems; identify appropriate modifications in sexual practices in response to these limitations; and report satisfying sexual activity.

Interventions:
- Assess for causative or contributing factors (e.g., decreased hormone production, fatigue, pain, depression, anxiety, medications [antidepressants, antihistamines, antihypertensives, chemotherapeutics, narcotics, sedatives], change in body image); assess for feelings of guilt associated with desiring touch and needing sexual activity, then assure the patient and partner that sexual expression, even when one has cancer, is natural and that need for intimacy often increases during this time.
- Assess for changes in role function and sexually defined gender roles; encourage discussion between partners about roles; encourage negotiation about role changes, which may be temporary.
- Assess for fear of being contagious; assure patient and partner that cancer cannot be transmitted through sexual activity.
- Assess for changes in body image, such as hair loss, and discuss alternatives.
- Assess for fatigue and explain that severe fatigue may hinder sexual desire but it does not indicate rejection of partner; encourage verbal and nonverbal communication between patient and partner.
- Assess for effects of alkylating agents, antimetabolites, and antitumor antibiotics, including decreased desire, ovarian dysfunction, and erectile dysfunction, and discuss changes in body appearance/function.
- Assess for effects of vinca alkaloids, including retrograde ejaculation, erectile dysfunction, decreased sexual desire or arousal, and ovarian dysfunction; encourage nonsexual touching, rest, and avoidance of alcoholic beverages, narcotics, and sedatives before sexual activity; suggest use of water-soluble lubricants to decrease vaginal irritation and avoidance of oral and anal sex during periods of neutropenia.
- Assess for side effects of radiation therapy, including fatigue, neutropenia, and anorexia; teach patient to plan sexual activity after rest periods and to use positions that require less exertion for the patient; encourage nonsexual touching and communication; remind patient and partner that patient is not radioactive while undergoing external-beam radiation treatment, and discuss site-specific side effects and their impact on sexual functioning.
- Explore patient's pattern of sexual functioning; encourage patient to share concerns and discuss the relationship between sexual functioning and stressors.
- Reaffirm the need for frank discussion between sexual partners; include need for closeness and expressions of caring through touching, massage, and other means; suggest that sexual

activity does not always culminate in vaginal intercourse but that the partner can reach orgasm through noncoital stimulation.

- Explain that attempting lovemaking while fatigued, while experiencing a chest infection, after a large meal, or after indulgence in large amounts of alcohol increases the likelihood of failure.
- Suggest that planned lovemaking during midday or early evening when energy levels are highest may be more satisfying than late-night relations when the patient is fatigued.
- Encourage adherence to the medical regimen to promote maximum recovery.
- Teach possible modification in sexual practices to assist in dealing with limitations caused by illness (e.g., modifications in positions, use of pillows for comfort and/or balance, techniques to control drainage or odor, use of clothing to cover affected body part).
- Provide referrals, if indicated, to an enterostomal therapist, physician, nurse specialist, or sex therapist.

Impaired Social Interactions Related to Embarrassment, Limited Physical Mobility, or Energy Secondary to Loss of Body Function or Terminal Illness

Definition: The state in which the patient experiences or is at risk of experiencing negative, insufficient, or unsatisfactory responses from interactions

Major defining characteristics: Inability to establish or maintain stable, supportive relationships; dissatisfaction with social network

Older adult considerations: Effective social interactions depend on positive self-esteem; no data suggest that older adults have diminished self-esteem compared with younger adults; common threats to self-esteem in older adults include devaluation, dependency, functional impairments, and decreased sense of control; depression-related affective disturbances of daily life occur in 27% of older adults, while major depression occurs in 2% of community-living older adults and in 12% of older people living in nursing homes (Parmelee, Katz, & Lawton, 1989); depressed older adults lose interest in social activities and do not display positive interactions when they do interact.

Outcome criteria: The patient will identify problematic behavior that deters socialization and substitute constructive behavior for disruptive social behavior; the family will describe strategies to promote effective socialization.

Interventions:

- Provide support for the maintenance of basic social skills and the reduction of social isolation or loneliness; assist the patient to manage life stresses; focus on the present and reality; identify how stress precipitates problems; support healthy defenses; identify alternative courses of action, and analyze approaches that work best; provide supportive group therapy if appropriate, for this person.
- Monitor medication compliance while assessing for side effects and exacerbation of symptoms.
- Be assertive with people who are unmotivated or passive.
- Use a variety of agencies and services, including medical, psychiatric, vocational, social, and residential; one agency or a case manager should coordinate services, and programs must be flexible and culturally relevant.
- *Note.* The new nursing diagnosis of "Loneliness," which is in the developmental process, might more accurately describe this situation and should be considered when it is fully developed by the North American Nursing Diagnosis Association.

Spiritual Distress Related to Challenge to Belief System or Separation From Spiritual Ties Secondary to Terminal Illness, Debilitating Disease, Pain, or Loss of Body Function

Definition: The state in which the patient experiences or is at risk of experiencing a disturbance in the belief or value system that provides strength, hope, and meaning to life

Major defining characteristic: Experiences a disturbance in belief system

Older adult considerations: Factors that contribute to spiritual distress and put older adults at risk include questions concerning life after death as the person ages, separation from formal religious community, and a value-belief system that is continuously challenged by losses and suffering; prayer, a common coping method for older adults, increases feelings of self-worth and hope by reducing the sense of aloneness and abandonment; older adults can counterbalance some of the negative and isolating aspects of aging by identifying with tradition and institutional values; private religion can help to motivate and provide purpose to life; older adults commonly intertwine their religious beliefs with beliefs about health and illness; older adults commonly report a sense of increased power and control from religion and spiritual resources; in one study, approximately 25% of older adults in nursing homes reported that a nurse had helped them with their spiritual needs, although 79% were against nursing involvement in their spiritual lives because of differing beliefs and a concern that the nurse needed to focus on physical care (Post-White et al., 1996).

Outcome criteria: The patient will express feelings related to change in beliefs, describe spiritual belief system positively, express desire to perform religious/spiritual practices, and describe satisfaction with meaning and purpose of illness, suffering, and death.

Interventions:
- Assess for causative and contributing factors, such as failure of spiritual beliefs, to provide explanation or comfort during crisis of illness, suffering, or impending death and anger toward God or spiritual beliefs for allowing or causing illness, suffering, or death.
- Eliminate or reduce causative and contributing factors, if possible.
- Suggest using prayer, imagery, and meditation to view self as a survivor rather than as a victim.
- Communicate concerns seriously by being available to listen to the patient's feelings and questions.
- Give "permission" to discuss spiritual matters.
- Offer to contact usual or new spiritual leader.
- Offer to pray, meditate, or read with patient, if comfortable, or arrange for someone else to do so if more appropriate.
- Provide uninterrupted quiet time for prayer, reading, or meditation.
- Employ silence and/or touch in communicating presence and support during times of doubt or despair.
- Suggest process of "life review" to identify past sources of strength or spiritual support.
- Express to patient that anger toward God is a common reaction to illness, suffering, or death.
- Help patient to recognize and discuss feelings of anger.
- Offer to contact another spiritual support person (e.g., pastoral care, hospital chaplain, social worker) if patient cannot share feelings with usual spiritual leader.

See Chapter 12 for an in-depth discussion of spirituality and the older adult with cancer.

Conclusion

Nursing diagnoses and interventions can be implemented after an assessment of the QOL of the older patient with cancer. The COOP Charts, supplemented here, are well suited for clinical assessment of QOL for older adults with cancer. They provide a reliable, valid means of assessing the physical, psychosocial, and spiritual realms of a person's life. They have been tested on elderly patients and have been found to be valid with this population. The charts can be briefly administered by nursing clinicians and support staff, or they can be self-administered by the patient. Patient understanding of the charts is supported by preparation of the charts at an eighth-grade reading level, which can accommodate most of the older adults in American society. Visual representations that assist those with a lower reading level or those who have mild cognitive impairment also are included. In addition, the charts are available in several languages other than English.

As Bennahum et al. (1997) noted, balancing cure and care is an important concept in the treatment of people of all ages who have cancer, but it is especially relevant for older adults with cancer. Cure may not be possible for many. Therefore, medical treatments must be balanced with support for and caring of the patient by family, friends, and healthcare providers. The gerontologic nurse and oncology nurse can provide those elements of care through the use of a nursing process that can make the difference in the patient's quality of life.

References

Bennahum, D.A., Forman, W.B., Vellas, B., & Albarede, J.L. (1997). Life expectancy, comorbidity, and quality of life: A framework of reference for medical decisions. *Clinics in Geriatric Medicine, 13*(1), 33–53.

Bland, K.I. (1997). Quality-of-life management for cancer patients. *CA: A Cancer Journal for Clinicians, 47*, 194–197.

Capra, F. (1996). *The web of life: A new scientific understanding of living systems.* New York: Doubleday.

Carpenito, L.J. (1997). *Nursing diagnosis: Application to clinical practice* (7th ed.). Philadelphia: Lippincott.

Cella, D.F., & Bonomi, A.E. (1995). Measuring quality of life: 1995 update. *Oncology, 9*(Suppl. 11), 47–60.

Eliopoulos, C. (1995). *Gerontological nursing* (2nd ed.). Philadelphia: Lippincott.

Gralla, R.J., & Moinpour, C.M. (1995). *Assessing quality of life in patients with lung cancer: A guide for clinicians.* New York: NCM Publishers.

King, C.R., Haberman, M., Berry, D.L., Bush, N., Butler, L., Dow, K.H., Ferrell, B., Grant, M., Gue, D., Hinds, P., Kreuer, J., Padilla, G., & Underwood, S. (1997). Quality of life and the cancer experience: The state-of-the-knowledge. *Oncology Nursing Forum, 24*, 27–41.

Nelson, E.C., Landgraf, J.M., Hayes, R.D., Wasson, J., & Kirk, J.W. (1990). The functional status of patients. How can it be measured in physicians' offices? *Medical Care, 28*, 1111–1126.

Nelson, E.C., Wasson, J., Kirk, J., Keller, A., Clark, D., Dietrich, A., Stewart, A., & Zubkoff, M. (1987). Assessment of function in routine clinical practice: Description of the COOP chart method and preliminary findings. *Journal of Chronic Diseases, 40*(Suppl. 1), 55S–63S.

Parmelee, P.A., Katz, I.R., & Lawton, M.P. (1989). Depression among institutionalized aged. *Journal of Gerontology: Medical Sciences, 44*(1), 22–29.

Post-White, J., Ceronsky, C., Kreitzer, M.J., Nickelson, K., Drew, D., Mackey, K.W., Koopmeiners, L., & Gutknecht, S. (1996). Hope, spirituality, sense of coherence, and quality of life in patients with cancer. *Oncology Nursing Forum, 23*, 1571–1578.

Siu, A.L., Hays, R.D., Ouslander, J.G., Osterwell, D., Valdez, R.B., Krynski, M., & Gross, A. (1993). Measuring functioning and health in the very old. *Journal of Gerontology Medical Sciences, 48*(1), M10–M14.

Turner, S. (1997). Quality-adjusted life years: Cost effective medical decision-making. *Journal of Oncology Management, 6*(4), 30–34.

Trustees of Dartmouth College. (1996). *Dartmouth COOP project.* Hanover, NH: The COOP Project.

Chapter Twelve

Spiritual Care of the Older Adult With Cancer

Sandra Skorupa, RN, MS

Introduction

Nursing originated in religious orders, where the body and spirit were cared for simultaneously. However, about a century ago, the philosophy of care began to move away from a holistic toward a dualistic approach. Focus on the care of the body increased, while the importance of care of the spirit declined over time. The rapid growth of technological advances in medicine, which produced inflation in healthcare costs, had a dramatic impact on this shift. As medical specialties were on the rise, the dominos continued to fall with the issues of the uninsured, malpractice/insurance costs, and increasing regulatory constraints. These factors all continue to pressure the movement of managed care as acute-care facilities struggle to meet the needs of the poor while maintaining a healthy financial bottom line and compliance with the Joint Commission on Accreditation of Healthcare Organizations (JCAHO), Department of Health, and other regulatory standards. Consequently, nursing remains dominated by the medical model despite attempts to rediscover holism through the incorporation of complementary therapies.

The foundation of nursing practice continues to be rooted in the promotion of wellness and the achievement of optimum health potential. As nurses learn early in nursing school, high-level wellness requires the integration of the whole being of the person—mind, body, and spirit. Older adults, in particular, are at risk of experiencing diminished levels of wellness or wholeness. While physical functioning may be at risk, the spiritual dimension of life remains an essential element of the total human being. The spiritual quest can be undertaken as completely by an atheist or agnostic, or a worshiper of nature, family, mankind, art, music, or science, as by a believer in an explicitly religious or spiritual tradition. Therefore, spirituality can positively influence the health of older adults and should be incorporated into effective nursing care management.

The Spiritual Dimension

Spirituality can be described as the central artery that diffuses throughout and vitalizes all other dimensions of an individual. Many people believe that without spiritual well-being, the biopsychosocial dimension cannot function. Therefore, spiritual health is vital to optimum quality of life. While the biopsychosocial dimension can be described with a reasonable degree of clarity, the spiritual dimension is a much more complex and personal concept. Due to this ambiguity, definitions vary slightly among experts. However, a goal of this chapter is to provide a well-rounded, fundamental understanding of the spiritual dimension.

Intrinsic Religiosity

Intrinsic religiosity is a construct similar to spiritual well-being, which is the terminology used by the National Interfaith Coalition on Aging to mean "the affirmation of life in a relationship with God, self, community, and environment that nurtures and celebrates wholeness" (Mullen, Smith, & Hill, 1993, p. 26). Spiritual well-being has been conceptualized as two-faceted. It encompasses a vertical dimension, or one's sense of well-being in relation to God, and a horizontal dimension, or one's sense of life purpose and satisfaction (Mullen et al.).

Renetzky, as discussed in Ross (1995), provided a definition that probably best captures and summarizes the spiritual dimension, which consists of three components.
1. The "power within man," giving "meaning, purpose, and fulfillment" to life, suffering, and death
2. The individual's "will to live"
3. The individual's belief and faith in self, others, and God

Human beings are driven to search for the ultimate meaning and purpose of their lives. Jung and Peck, respectively, postulated that meaning is necessary for the maintenance of ego integrity and for the prevention of restlessness and deterioration in old age (Ross, 1995). Throughout the cancer experience, the patient's ability to invest life with meaning is continuously challenged as each milestone is reached or a positive prognosis is threatened.

The will to live, hope, and cope is interrelated and contingent in the promotion of healing. Consequently, death can be anticipated as an outcome of helplessness/hopelessness and may be considered "passive suicide." Ross (1995) discussed the premise that the greater the will to live, the greater the chance the patients had of overcoming illness.

While healthy individuals can initiate actions to meet their own spiritual needs, older adults with cancer, as well as their support systems, may experience spiritual distress stemming from the effects of the cancer diagnosis and its meaning. Illness and hospitalization cause some people to face loss of control for the first time in their lives. Questions may outnumber answers, and some may never be answered to satisfaction. Some patients with cancer feel enriched and supported by their faith, while others may feel robbed and abandoned, which often prompts a negative confrontation with the concept of a loving God.

Organized Religion

Organized religious activity is, by far, the most common form of voluntary social participation practiced by older adults in this country (Koenig, Larson, & Matthews, 1996). However, the regularity of church attendance is not always directly related to the depth of a meaningful belief system. Some patients feel comforted through religious beliefs, while others feel abandoned. According to a national survey, 61% of older people read the Bible weekly or more often, 95% pray (88% pray alone), and 58% watch religious television programming (Koenig et al.). Finally, the personal dimension of religious involvement, indicated by strength of belief, importance of religion, and intrinsic religiosity, is widespread among the elderly, with more than 75% of people age 65 or older indicating that religion is very important to them (Koenig et al.). In a review of nearly 100 studies, Koenig et al. found that religiously committed older adults who frequently attended church, prayed, or read religious books were healthier, happier, and more satisfied with their lives and were less depressed, anxious, lonely, or likely to abuse alcohol than less religiously committed elders. Religious beliefs and practices are notably more prevalent among the older adult population, and 95% of older Americans practice from a Judeo-Christian tradition (Koenig et al.). One study determined a positive relationship between age and spirituality, supporting the theoretical view of spirituality as developing through life as another dimension of human experience (Ita, 1995–1996).

Coping

Many elders use religion as a coping behavior to help them to deal with potentially disabling mental and physical disorders. When older people were asked a direct question about whether or not they use religion as a coping strategy, almost 90% responded affirmatively (Koenig et al., 1996). Even when asked open-ended questions about their coping strategies (without mentioning religion), 24%–40% of older adults spontaneously offered religious responses, especially women and minority elders (Koenig et al.). However, the question remains whether religious behaviors truly enhance coping effectiveness. Little research has focused on the role of spiritual resources as a mediating variable between stressful events and adaptational outcomes. One illustration of the differences and complexities in approaches to coping with a single religious group involved a sample drawn from Protestant denominations. The subjects identified three distinct religious ways of maintaining a sense of organization and control in coping.
1. "Collaborative" religious coping—God was defined as a partner who shared responsibility with the individual for problem solving.
2. "Deferring" coping—Responsibility was delegated to God while passively waiting for the outcome.
3. "Self-directed" coping—Assumption that God has provided the skills and resources for independent problem solving (Jenkins & Pargament, 1995).
Later, a fourth approach was identified based on attempts to influence the will of God by praying for recovery or pleading for a miracle.

In the research and clinical realms, spirituality tends to be viewed as a passive way of coping or as a defense mechanism. Consequently, the impact of spirituality on effective coping often is misunderstood and is not given credence. However, evidence exists to support religion as part of an active coping style in patients who have an internal locus of control and associated high levels of personal competence and the ability to initiate problem solving.

The goal of coping is resolution of a problem. Older adults bring a lifelong history of coping to the point of initial cancer diagnosis. Positive coping strategies can be identified when the patient with cancer exhibits specific behaviors. Through nurse-patient interactions, the desired goal in the plan of care should be reality confrontation with minimal avoidance behaviors.

Open and mutual communication is critical among all significant parties involved. The nurse must recognize behaviors of ineffective coping, which may include powerlessness, low self-esteem, and self-deception. As a result, signs of ineffective coping may present as withdrawal, suppression, substance abuse, passive acceptance, and impulsive, risky behaviors. The assistance of an advanced practice nurse, social worker, or physician may be warranted at this point.

Coping is supported not only by negative feelings, such as anger, denial, or depression, but also by enhancement of positive feelings. The natural feeling of hope that a patient with cancer has is a valuable asset in the promotion of the ability to cope.

Hope

As a focal point, hope can provide the necessary balance for the practitioner when the tendency is to focus on negative behaviors. Callan (1989) noted that an entire chapter in *On Death and Dying* (Kübler-Ross, 1969) was devoted to hope. The chapter began as follows: "We have discussed so far the different stages that people go through when they are faced with tragic news. . . . The one thing that usually persists through all these stages is hope" (p. 138).

The concept of hope is highly personal and, therefore, can be difficult to comprehend. Definitions of hope include emotions, expectations, illusions, and disposition. It has been characterized as having two distinct focuses. An optimistic view of life or the world is described as generalized hope. In comparison, particularized hope is defined as hope that is directed toward a specific outcome with personal meaning.

In a study addressing the relationship between hope and caring in individuals who have been diagnosed with cancer, researchers found a positive correlation between hope and effective coping (McCray, 1997). Hopefulness has an impact on the ability to function independently in self-care or maintain a responsible role in the family; it generally is facilitated by a strong religious faith. An effective nurse-patient-family relationship is critical to the ability to assess false hope and maladaptive denial.

Hope for the future can be the universal hope for a cure or more attainable hopes, such as to leave the hospital soon, achieve a remission, attend a significant family event, or be free of pain. The importance of these hopes should be prioritized as significant in the care of older adults. All healthcare providers have a role in supporting patients' ability to hope, as well as in working with family members and significant others to do the same.

Pain

Studies have demonstrated relationships between spirituality and decreased levels of pain, anxiety, hostility, and social isolation as well as higher levels of life satisfaction and lower mortality rates in patients with cancer (Jenkins & Pargament, 1995). Cancer pain places demands on the spiritual dimension, resulting in distress that can threaten patients' perception of wholeness. Spiritual distress occurs because the harmony of the mind, body, and spirit is disrupted. Nurses must assist patients to promote control over pain and diminish the physical distress related to living with advanced or recurrent cancer. Effective pain-management strategies integrate direct care, effective use of medications, teaching, counseling, alternative healing modalities (e.g., therapeutic touch, music therapy), and social support, including augmentation by case managers and community resources. As with most nursing interventions, a comprehensive approach in the plan of care yields positive outcomes.

The meaning of cancer pain also is a significant consideration in the nurse-patient relationship. According to Georgesen and Dungan (1996), patients equated increasing intensity of pain with disease progression. Patients equated dying with the inability to achieve pain relief and experienced loss of independence, control, and usefulness. Holistic pain management by the nurse, in collaboration with the patient, family, and caregivers, is clearly implicated. Spiritual awareness can promote comforting personal perspectives on death with less psychosocial distress. Consequently, hospice programs that focus on a holistic approach to patient-centered nursing care have embraced this philosophy.

Nursing Implications

Assessment of spiritual well-being clearly is within the domain of nursing. The JAREL Spiritual Well-Being Scale is an assessment tool used in establishing nursing diagnoses regarding spirituality in older adults (Hungelmann, Kenkel-Rossi, Klassen, & Stollenwerk, 1996). The JAREL Spiritual Well-Being Scale is a 21-item Likert-type scale that incorporates the broad dimensions of spiritual well-being. Through factor analysis, the researchers identified three factors associated with subsets of seven questions.

- The faith/belief dimension
- Life/self-responsibility
- Life satisfaction/self-actualization

If a patient's score on an item, group of items, or particular factor is low, it may identify a need for further investigation or follow-up. The patient has a relationship with spiritual well-being core categories, and properties identified as outcomes in this study are as follows (Hungelmann et al., 1996).

- Ultimate Other (believes in Supreme Being, trust in, God, etc.)
- Other/nature (accepts/gives help, expresses mutual love, etc.)
- Self (values inner self, has a positive attitude, etc.)
- Time
  - Past (expresses growth/change over time, recognizes parental influences, etc.)
  - Present (lives up to potential, is open to change, etc.)
  - Future (sets goals, searches for meaning/purpose in life, etc.).

Nursing Research

Nursing research on spiritual care in older adults with cancer is very much in its infancy. One could infer that nurses' provision of spiritual care is poor, infrequent, or even nonexistent. Nursing issues that have an impact on spiritual care include narrow conceptualization, fear of incompetence, uncertainty regarding personal values and beliefs, and discomfort with the circumstances that prompt the identification of spiritual needs. These issues are consistent with those of other healthcare professionals, particularly physicians. In addition, nurses may not believe that spiritual care is within the domain of nursing (Taylor, Amenta, & Highfield, 1995); this also is consistent with the medical model.

Practicing nurses are aware that patients have spiritual needs, and many recognize their responsibility and express the desire to be involved in meeting these needs. However, nurses typically feel that they are unable to provide spiritual care adequately and, in fact, recognize the need for further education. This need for education must be addressed if gerontologic and oncologic nursing are to continue to evolve in the areas of complementary medicine and palliative care. As we rethink nursing credentialing requirements, the concept of "spiritual competence" needs to be added if our goals are to include "caring for the soul."

The Physician's Role

Historically, spirituality and medicine were as easily intertwined as the snake and caduceus symbolizing the healing arts. While modern mainstream medicine traditionally has been skeptical about faith and healing, the integration of faith into treatment plans can be observed in current practice. Studies of patient-physician interaction and the role that spirituality plays in these encounters primarily are focused on the specialties of oncology, geriatrics, and psychiatry. Physician exploration into religious issues tends to be rare and specific to serious or life-threatening events. It has been suggested that physicians do not address spiritual needs because of a lack of awareness of their importance, personal discomfort with the subject matter, or a fear of imposing their own personal beliefs (Daaleman & Nease, 1994). A study of patient attitudes regarding physician inquiry into spiritual and religious issues identified a consistent finding that physicians should refer patients with spiritual problems to clergy or other professionals trained in this area (Daaleman & Nease). Unfortunately, physician referral patterns to the clergy have been minimally studied; Koenig et al. (1996) briefly mentioned that fewer than one-half of the physicians they surveyed reported a pattern of referral to the clergy when their elderly patients were near death or experiencing great distress. Four contributing factors include the absence of religious beliefs, lack of availability of appropriate clergy, assumption that religious patients will self-refer and that nonreligious patients have no desire for this intervention, and lack of knowledge specific to utilization/benefits of clergy in a clinical situation. Physicians need to understand that patients want to be cured of their disease, but they refocus their goals when they accept that hope for cure is not realistic. When cure is impossible, care is essential (Spiegel, 1995).

The Role of Social Workers and Other Healthcare Professionals

Because social workers, as laypeople, sometimes can deal more easily with patients' spiritual issues than chaplains can, it is important to view this role as appropriate for social workers (Carr & Morris, 1996). Similar to nurses and physicians, social workers may avoid discussing spiritual issues because they view the subject as too personal and feel inadequately trained in this area. In this era of shorter hospital stays, increased patient acuity, and briefer interactions between healthcare professionals and patients, the identification of the ability to cope can be particularly useful in managing care. The personal spiritual beliefs of the social worker are important. "Nonbelievers may not be fully able to accept clients who consider spirituality and religion to be meaningful and useful within the context of their life experiences" (Sermabeikian, 1994, pp. 178–179). Social workers often make referrals to hospital chaplains, patients' pastors, or other spiritual leaders. However, social workers may provide more effective interventions than clergy because of their ability to project a nonjudgmental attitude. Some patients may be more comfortable approaching social workers than members of the religious community. Finally, timing can be an issue, particularly with patients who have terminal disease and could die before clergy can be accessed. In these circumstances, social workers can certainly address spiritual concerns.

The Role of the Clergy

The clergy's role in the healthcare environment needs to be recognized as vital in both the care of patients with cancer and their families and in the support of all healthcare professionals rather than focusing primarily on end-of-life decision making in the hospital setting. To meet this need, the clergy must become better prepared for the entry of science into practice. Although relationships exist between prayer and religious devotion and positive health outcomes, those in the religious sector still may not consistently adopt this belief. Even true believers often doubt, at some level, the effectiveness of prayer, and religious professionals may be shocked to discover that science has something positive to say about prayer (Dossey, 1997). Those who have been educated and socialized in 20th-century America tend to understand only two approaches to living. We can be intellectual, rational, and scientific or intuitive, spiritual, and religious. In the past, these two opposing approaches were viewed as incompatible. The future trend, however, is to unite spirituality and science, which naturally requires a shift in thinking by both religious and healthcare professionals. A vision of chaplaincy and education for the 21st century includes four characteristics specific to the delivery of spiritual-care needs: the ability to address spirituality in a geographic, community-based, coordinated, and integrated manner. A clearer definition of the new chaplain is emerging. Charting, spiritual assessment, case conferences, interdisciplinary teaming, and ethical counseling have brought chaplains closer to their allied professionals, but they need to grow closer still (Driscoll, 1995).

Psychological and Spiritual Needs of Older Adults

Spiritual Needs

Spiritual needs stem from a conscious awareness that life is finite and that people are called to a higher purpose. Significant overlap exists between spiritual and psychological needs, and together they produce a complete picture of human need. To illustrate these needs, a discussion of nine psychological and spiritual needs of older adults follows.

Meaning, Purpose, and Hope

Elderly people can grow and continually develop a philosophy that gives life meaning. Healthy aging adults, faced with all of the expected personal and social losses, experience coping struggles with normal, everyday life. As families with children of their own increasingly are caring for aging parents, as well, evidence of this growth and development crisis can be seen in the average American household. The search for meaning, purpose, and hope is challenged further as older adults are forced to cope with progressive health problems, pain, and disability. As a result, older adults turn to God for inner strength and positive perspective. These roads to inner peace can provide support to struggling older adults with cancer.

Transcendence

A cancer diagnosis immediately conjures up images of increasing disability, suffering, and the threat of eventual death, particularly in older adults. This reality usually is overwhelming, particularly at the onset, and can forecast the reality of a dismal future. Religious faith can provide the ability to overcome, or transcend, these difficult life circumstances.

Self-Esteem and Respect

So much of who we are revolves around our accomplishments, relationships, and social roles. Aging, complicated by cancer, can threaten this identity and self-esteem and cause profound lifestyle changes. A spiritual view of the world can help an individual to make sense out of loss and suffering. Spiritual beliefs provide a mechanism of control at a time when life feels totally out of control.

Life Review

As people age and are faced with a multitude of losses, they begin to analyze life and its meaning. This life review can be very satisfying—or it can be devastating. The outcome produced is the major psychosocial crisis in the final stage of life, integrity versus despair. Again, while healthy adults face these normal life crises, older adults with cancer perceive these struggles with intensified vulnerability. Religious beliefs can promote new beginnings through forgiving and forgetting of the past and focus on future changes.

Religious Faith: Private and Public

Older adults need the opportunity and time for prayer and reading, as well as to be able to attend public worship as long as possible. These activities nurture the elder's spirit and may facilitate improved clinical outcomes, as previous research has shown (Koenig et al., 1996). However, this need is particularly challenged in home- or hospital-bound elders who wish to attend religious services. Television services or visits by a parish nurse or member of the clergy may provide an acceptable substitute.

Anger, Questions, and Uncertainty

"Why me?" is a question asked at some point by every patient diagnosed with cancer. The human tendency is to rationalize and attach blame to any perceived inequity in life. When bad things happen to good people, the natural reaction is to hold God responsible. Temporary alienation from God has an impact on coping ability, produces guilt, and interferes with the healing process. Older adults need the opportunity and permission to vent these feelings, reassurance that these feelings are normal, and a chance to work through them. The expertise of the clergy may be very beneficial at this time in terms of counseling or the provision of a religious sacrament.

Love and Service

The basic human need to love and reach out to others is compromised by cancer in elderly adults. The ability to provide service to the church and community can be very important and satisfying to those in this particular age group. The role of caregivers may be to identify creative solutions that will allow homebound older adults to meet this need (e.g., contact other shut-ins who need support, complete arts-and-crafts projects or baking to donate to a church or community fund-raiser). In meeting this need, elders may begin to reestablish their sense of worth through these new achievements. As a result, prior losses are replaced and self-esteem is enhanced.

Expression of Appreciation

One of the most powerful human needs is the need to be thankful, which is reflected repeatedly in both Old and New Testament verses. Personal well-being and mental health have a close relationship to the ability to meet this need. As older adults face cancer, a potentially life-threatening illness, it is natural to focus on the negative aspects and the feeling of being cheated of life. Spiritual and emotional well-being are threatened with this attitude. Because thankfulness can be a learned behavior acquired through practice, healthcare providers can assist patients by providing support, encouragement, and direction. The ability to be optimistic and focus on the "glass half-full" is unnatural for many people and must be cultivated.

Preparation for Death and Dying

An uncertain future pressures older adults to "put things in order." Through this life-review process, unresolved guilt, resentment, and regret for real and imagined sins may emerge.

Older adults rarely volunteer this information, which presents another opportunity for caregivers to intervene. They need forgiveness from God and from themselves, and spiritual rituals may be helpful in allowing this giving and receiving of forgiveness.

Religious beliefs and rituals (e.g., the sacrament of Extreme Unction or Sacrament of the Sick in the Catholic tradition) can be vital to ease fears and organize the dying process. Even though ministers, priests, or rabbis traditionally have been involved in this preparation process, these issues are likely to surface with caregivers, who can work with patients toward meeting this need.

This information equips caregivers with a basic understanding of patient and family needs in this area. One intervention may meet a multitude of needs or at least lay the foundation and establish the environment for progress in other areas. Spirituality needs to be a vital component of a comprehensive patient assessment and plan of care if nurses are to be effective in meeting the total needs of older patients with cancer. Spiritual competence may need to be incorporated into nursing education and orientation processes.

Wellness Spirituality in the Older Patient With Cancer

Nurses have the responsibility to create a spiritually nurturing environment in which to assess spiritual needs and manage older patients' plans of care. The timing of a spiritual assessment is vital to effective intervention. Although assessment is emphasized in the initial stages, it should be an ongoing task (Millison, 1995). To intervene effectively with older patients, attention must be paid to cultural factors. If cultural beliefs are not taken into account, the goals established may turn out to be irrelevant. For example, expecting a patient to transition from productive to leisure activities will occur only if the patient's culture supports this shift.

In thinking about the aging process, it is useful to consider three themes that run like threads throughout our lives. The physical thread, which peaks at age 21, focuses on the condition of our bodies and slowly and gradually declines. The economic thread, which peaks at age 40, deals with the condition of our economic and monetary wealth and our ability to make a living. The human thread, which measures our emergence as full people, continues to develop in older years and peaks only at the time of death. Unfortunately, we grow older in a culture that expects little from the elderly other than predictable decline and medical needs. The elderly are expected to fade and become less, which is only expedited with a diagnosis of cancer.

Nursing Interventions

Because many nurses do not feel adequately prepared to meet patients' spiritual needs, they must be equipped with resources to support this assessment and intervention. A patient-assessment process or tool might include questions specific to patients' responses to conditions in life or illness. For example, inquiries specific to disability, altered body image, chronic pain, anger toward others or God, isolation, or changes in meaningful relationships would be significant information for nurses. History taking regarding self-actualization activities (e.g., plans for the future, roles in family, coping), connectedness activities (e.g., staying in touch with significant others, support networks), healing and new life activities (e.g., meaning for life, the role of one's God), and religious and humanistic activities (e.g., relationship with the organized church, helpfulness of prayer, religious rituals, sacraments) create a comprehensive database from which to plan care and establish goals.

Utilizing outcomes of patients' assessments, nurses can develop a plan of care. In managing care effectively, nurses must consult or refer to the clergy, a spiritual leader, or a parish nurse when they recognize that spiritual needs require this level of expertise. The plan of care must address self-actualization. This goal can be met through supporting independence, teaching methods of visual imagery of life accomplishments, discussing anxieties about the future, and basic listening, support, and encouragement. The plan of care should work toward supporting and restoring connectedness. Creative strategies to meet this goal can include arranging mentorships or storytelling with adults or children, letter "writing" by tape to grandchildren, friends, or even politicians, and volunteering service when feasible. The plan of care needs to support or restore religious and humanistic activities orientation. This goal can be met through activities such as journal keeping, recycling, indoor gardening, prayer or meditation, and access to religious or spiritual articles and religious ceremonies.

The care model that supports spiritual wellness demands a shared community between practitioners and aging clients. Through this mutual bonding, nurses discover who these older adults really are while the aging patient reaches an understanding of "Why am I?" and "What is the meaning of my life?" Nurses need to demonstrate the virtues of hospitality, awareness, vulnerability, compassion, and commitment to produce effective patient outcomes. In effect, nurses need to be kind to the old person they will be some day.

Four Areas of Nursing Interventions

Four areas of nursing interventions include affirmation, therapeutic communication, reminiscence, and referral. As a follow-up to any patient assessment, nurses review the information obtained and identify the "gift" to be affirmed or the need to be met by listening to patients.

Through affirmation, a positive force in patients' lives may be identified that can be useful in providing effective spiritual care. In contrast, an area of spiritual distress may be identified, such as a strained relationship with a child in the case of the older adult. Nurses can work with patients on strategies to achieve inner peace.

Through therapeutic communication, nurses and patients explore areas of strength, pain, and loss. Nurses need to realize the value of silence and presence, which can be the most important skills they offer. Spiritual assessments provide a knowledge base of patients' spiritual well-being from which nurses can initiate discussion, depending upon the openness and cues offered by patients. Listening and observation are critical in planning spiritual care. Expressions and body language can provide helpful cues, which need to be validated prior to being acted upon.

The feeling of having lived a meaningful life is a common thread in the fabric of spiritual health. Consequently, it should be no surprise that reminiscence of meaningful past people, situations, or events with follow-up exploration is a process to be encouraged by nurses. Heliker (1995) identified that modified life review can be used as a guide in assessment, enabling patients and nurses to discover areas of strength as well as new possibilities in patients' lives. Areas of strengths, "brokenness," and unresolved feelings can emerge. Nurses and patients can then work toward strategies to resolve, let go of, or change any "unfinished business" in patients' lives.

The fourth intervention is initiated by nurses when responses indicate a negative perception on the part of patients and a referral to another healthcare professional or the clergy is indicated. This referral may be a welcomed relief, or it may not be desired at all. As with all healthcare interventions, patients are the ultimate decision makers. The role of the nurses as patient advocates is to always uphold the dignity of patients.

Reengineering Nursing Practice for the New Millennium

Arthur Koestler, in a bleak metaphor, called our time a "spiritual ice age" (Amenta & Bohnet, 1986). Fortunately, in the mid-1980s, the glaciers began to melt and today we live in a world of increasing spiritual orientation to life. However, creativity is critical to the reengineering of traditional interventional approaches to spiritual care. Understanding patients' coping styles and what nurtures their spirit is essential for the healing process. Because every spirit is nurtured in a very personal and unique way, it is vital that nurses complete an effective assessment through a comprehensive plan of care. One person's spirit may be nurtured by attendance at services and participation in community benefit activities, while another person may meet this need through music, art, or a nature walk. Older patients with cancer are empowered when they discover, or rediscover, this spiritual aspect of their lives. Nurses should be leaders in directing the healthcare team toward this goal. This is particularly important because, by the end of 2000, an estimated 100,000 Americans will have lived 100 years (Murphy & Hudson, 1995).

The increasing emphasis on patient rights also magnifies the need for spiritual care, particularly in the elderly oncology population for whom end-of-life decision making is increasingly prevalent. Advance directives and healthcare proxy have become standard agenda items at senior citizen gatherings. Pastoral-care services in the acute-care settings are experiencing increasing demand for support to patients and families in this decision-making process. The present dilemma is how to effectively equip nurses to meet spiritual-care needs for older patients with cancer and to integrate pastoral care into clinical care in both the acute and nonacute healthcare settings.

The healing process can be highly dependent upon spirituality in older patients with cancer. Nurses will continue to be faced with the challenge of meeting patients' biopsychosocial needs. The nursing profession will need to eliminate the "disease" associated with spiritual interventions. Caring for the whole person is the essence of nursing.

Hungelmann et al. (1996) discussed nursing icon Virginia Henderson's legacy as directing nurses to understand their unique function. That function included assisting well or sick people in the performance of daily activities. In this endeavor, nurses would contribute to the health or recovery or give support during the dying process to patients in a manner that provided care based on safeguarding the dignity of the individual.

Conclusion

The search for healing has always been the search for wholeness. The "being" of older patients with cancer emerges when the needs of the soul, as well as the body, are met. If life were a play, the last act would contain several surprises. Most significant would be that aging adults finally become in touch with the lightness of being, becoming more fully human than ever before. The human spirit grows to be more robust as the body becomes more frail. As a result, the spiritual mission of aging adults faced with a cancer diagnosis is to manage spiritual energy.

Limiting care to physical needs denies older patients meaningful and purposeful lives. Every nurse needs to recognize those moments when, through compassionate care, a difference has been made in patients' lives. Nurses who light the way in the uncertain journey of older patients with cancer will surely feel that the challenge and outcome of patient care was met.

References

Amenta, M.O., & Bohnet, N.L. (1986). *Nursing care of the terminally ill*. Boston: Little, Brown & Co.

Callan, D.B. (1989). Hope as a clinical issue in oncology social work. *Journal of Psychosocial Oncology, 7*(3), 31–46.

Carr, E.W., & Morris, T. (1996). Spirituality and patients with advanced cancer: A social work response. *Journal of Psychosocial Oncology, 14*(1), 71–81.

Daaleman, T.P., & Nease, D.E. (1994). Patient attitudes regarding physician inquiry into spiritual and religious issues. *Journal of Family Practice, 39*, 564–568.

Dossey, L. (1997). The return of prayer. *Alternative Therapies in Health and Medicine, 3*(6), 10–17, 113–120.

Driscoll, J.J. (1995). Courage for chaplaincy 2000. *Vision, 5*(4), 4–5.

Georgesen, J., & Dungan, J.M. (1996). Managing spiritual distress in patients with advanced cancer. *Cancer Nursing, 19*, 376–383.

Heliker, D. (1995). Personal meaning in the elderly: A Heideggerian hermeneutical phenomenological study. *Dissertation Abstracts International, 56*, 171B.

Hungelmann, J., Kenkel-Rossi, E., Klassen, L., & Stollenwerk, R. (1996). Focus on spiritual well-being: Harmonious interconnectedness of mind-body-spirit—Use of the JAREL spiritual well-being scale. *Geriatric Nursing, 17*, 262–266.

Ita, D.J. (1995–1996). Testing of a causal model: Acceptance of death in hospice patients. *Omega—Journal of Death and Dying, 32*(2), 81–91.

Jenkins, R.A., & Pargament, K.I. (1995). Religion and spirituality as resources for coping with cancer. *Journal of Psychosocial Oncology, 13*, 51–74.

Koenig, H.G., Larson, D.B., & Matthews, D.A. (1996). Religion and psychotherapy with older adults. *Journal of Geriatric Psychiatry, 29*, 155–184.

Kübler-Ross, E. (1969). *On death and dying*. New York: MacMillan.

McCray, N.D. (1997). Psychosocial and quality-of-life issues. In S.E. Otto (Ed.), *Oncology nursing* (3rd ed.) (pp. 817–834). St. Louis: Mosby.

Millison, M.B. (1995). A review of the research on spiritual care and hospice. *Hospice Journal, 10*(4), 3–18.

Mullen, P.M., Smith, R.M., & Hill, E.W. (1993). Sense of coherence as a mediator of stress for cancer patients and spouses. *Journal of Psychosocial Oncology, 11*(3), 23–46.

Murphy, J.S., & Hudson, F.M. (1995). *The joy of old*. Altadena, CA: Goede Press.

Ross, L. (1995). The spiritual dimension: Its importance to patient's health, well-being and quality of life and its implications for nursing practice. *International Journal of Nursing Studies, 32*, 457–468.

Sermabeikian, P. (1994). Our clients, ourselves: The spiritual perspective and social work practice. *Social Work, 39*(2), 178–183.

Spiegel, D. (1995). Commentary. *Journal of Psychosocial Oncology, 13*(1/2), 115–121.

Taylor, E.J., Amenta, M., & Highfield, M. (1995). Spiritual care practices of oncology nurses. *Oncology Nursing Forum, 22*, 31–39.

Chapter Thirteen

Legal Issues in Cancer Nursing
of the Older Adult

Alice G. Rini, JD, MS, RN

Definitions and Concepts Related to Law

Legal issues have become a major factor in nursing practice, regardless of the clinical specialty. Common expectations exist in terms of understanding the laws that govern practice, knowledge of legal principles, and expected standards to which nurses must adhere to avoid liability for malpractice. When nurses make clinical decisions that are the basis of patient care, they must at least ensure that

1. Such decisions are consistent with the law as it is currently interpreted.
2. They avoid liability for improper practice.
3. Patients are protected from harm.
   Law comes from a variety of sources: constitutions, which are the highest source of legal guidance; legislation, the written law promulgated by legislators, courts, and judges, which is the common law; and administrative law, which is the rules and regulations adopted by administrative agencies (Trandel-Korenchuk & Trandel-Korenchuk, 1997).

Standards of Practice in
Oncology Nursing of Older Adults

Standards of practice are found in nurse practice acts, which are legal documents promulgated by state boards of nursing as delegated by state legislatures, and in professional standards of practice, developed by professional organizations.

Nurse Practice Acts

Nursing practice is governed by state law. The law states what the practice of nursing should be and the knowledge and behavior expected of the practicing nurse. The standards mandated by nurse practice acts are required behaviors. Failure to adhere to such standards is grounds for license suspension or even revocation. Hearings to determine whether practice standards have been violated are held by the state's board of nursing, usually with its attorney prosecuting the accused nurse. Nurses who are subjects of investigation or who are summoned for hearings also should be represented by attorneys who are experienced in negotiating with professional boards. Such representation should begin when nurses first become aware that they have has been notified by the board of any charge. Standards set by boards of nursing are general in nature and usually do not refer to any particular nursing specialty.

Nurses also are subject to other laws that relate to patient relationships, communication, continuing-education requirements (in some states), reporting of abuse, and providing certain services through publicly supported programs. These laws, too, are general in nature and must be understood and applied in specific areas of practice in which nurses work.

Professional Standards of Practice

The American Nurses Association (ANA) developed the best known and most generally accepted standards of practice. Specialty groups promulgated standards specific to their area of practice from a general standards list (ANA, 1973, 1985). Important to the efforts of nurses caring for older adults with cancer are the *Standards and Scope of Gerontological Nursing Practice* (ANA, 1995) and the *Statement on the Scope and Standards of Oncology Nursing Practice* (ANA & Oncology Nursing Society, 1996).

Special Legal Issues in the Care of Older Adults With Cancer

Diagnostic Measures

Standard screening tests for common cancers are important diagnostic measures for early diagnosis, which is one of the most effective ways of preventing cancer deaths. However, some major policy and legal issues exist with regard to diagnostic tests.

Medicare will not pay for some diagnostic tests if no existing sign or symptom prompts their administration. Recently, screening mammograms for women and prostate-specific antigen (PSA) tests for men have been added to the list of Medicare-covered services. Other tests, however, are still not covered. Fecal occult blood tests are not covered even though colon cancer is one of the more common cancers of older adults. Some Medicare managed-care organizations cover more diagnostic tests than traditional Medicare, but some do not.

An interesting legal issue with regard to diagnostic testing is related to informed consent or, more specifically, informed refusal. When a patient refuses simple, low-risk diagnostic tests, whether covered by insurance or not, it is important to inform him or her about the risks and possible negative outcomes of avoiding the test and delaying a diagnosis. One court found a physician negligent for failing to *adequately* inform a woman about the risks of refusing a Pap test for cervical cancer (*Truman v. Thomas*, 1980). The woman later died from cervical cancer. Some evidence indicated that she refused the test because she could not afford it. Although the physician offered to defer payment, the patient still refused it. The *Truman* court also indicated that because the physician knew that undiagnosed cervical cancer was life-threatening, he had a duty to fully inform the patient of the significant risk of refusing the test even if he thought such information was well known by the general public. Interestingly, three of the California Supreme Court justices in the *Truman* case dissented from the majority. The dissenting argument noted that this verdict mandated an extensive educational program for patients who are deciding whether or not to undergo diagnostic tests; the justices indicated that such a program, even if justifiable, requires public policy to determine whether the cost warrants the burden and whether the duty to educate rests with doctors, schools, or health departments. Requiring individual doctors to be responsible for educating the public may be found to be an inefficient process that does not reach those who need it the most—the ones hesitant to consult doctors. Justice Clark, one of the dissenters, indicated that he believed that when a patient's doctor prescribes diagnostic tests, the patient is aware that the tests are intended to discover illness. It is reasonable to assume that a patient who refuses advice is aware of the potential risk.

Treatment Choices and Decisions About Treatment

Medicare may constrain treatment choices for older adults with cancer. Most decisions about reimbursement for health and medical care are made by local intermediaries, the public and private organizations that are contracted by the Department of Health and Human Services (DHHS) of the federal government to process Medicare claims. These agencies also have the power to determine what therapies will be covered. They are expected to use the scientific literature, local practice data, national databases, and industrial/medical sources, but a lack of uniformity and consistency exists in local practices, making it difficult to predict, particularly in the area of new technologies, which may be common in cancer care (Rosenblatt, Law, & Rosenbaum, 1997).

Managed Care

Managed care affects choices about treatment and the quality of that treatment. The DHHS has been attempting to encourage Medicare recipients to enroll in Medicare managed-care programs. A DHHS report (Brown, 1995) found pervasive quality problems throughout managed-care programs for Medicare, including difficulties in getting access to care; such quality problems already were observed in the private sector (Goodman & Musgrave, 1992). Managed-care organizations are less likely to use such diagnostic tests as magnetic resonance imaging (MRI) and computerized tomography (CT) scans. Both patients and healthcare providers have become dissatisfied. A 1988 survey by the American Medical Association (AMA) found that one-third of physicians expressed that patients were harmed by delays and nontreatment under managed care (Bandow & Tanner, 1995). Because Medicare spends four times as much on patients who die compared to those who live, it is likely that there is a great deal of pressure to save money by denying treatment to patients who are believed to be terminally ill. However, some research shows that physicians' predictions about who is terminally ill and who is not often are wrong (Bandow & Tanner).

Informed Consent

The legal doctrine of informed consent requires the disclosure of information about a proposed test or treatment that might be material to the patient's decision to accept or undergo the test or treatment. The information must be provided to the patient prior to obtaining consent. For consent to be truly informed, the information provided should (or must, as some courts have indicated) include the following (*Canterbury v. Spence*, 1972; Meisel & Kabnick, 1980; *Natanson v. Kline*, 1960).

- The diagnosis, including the tests and diagnostic procedures needed or used in its determination, alternatives to such tests, and the risks inherent in the procedures
- The nature and purpose of the proposed treatment
- The risks of treatment, including common and foreseeable risks
- The probability of success in cure, remission, or time to live; statistical information is appropriate, as well as the healthcare provider's experience with the procedure.
- Treatment alternatives generally considered feasible in practice; a caveat here is to be aware of the increasing popularity and some real success with the so-called "alternative" and "complementary" therapies, which are increasingly being integrated with the more common cancer therapies. In fact, cancer is the most frequently treated illness using these therapies.
- Prognosis with and without treatment

Informed consent is supported by the Patient Self-Determination Act (1991), which requires all healthcare institutions and agencies to

- Have written policies that provide adult patients the opportunity to consent to or refuse treatment.
- Inform patients concerning their rights under the state's law, including the right to make advance directives and other decisions regarding treatment and nontreatment.
- Assess for the existence of any advance directives and document them in the medical record.
- Not condition the provision of care on the basis of the presence or absence of an advance directive.
- Comply with state law concerning advance directives.
- Provide educational programs to agency staff and the community on the law and advance directives.

In the care of older adults with cancer, informed consent has some particularly important considerations.

Age of the patient: Age is important because there is some concern about the pervasive "ageism" in society. Assumptions are made about what older adults want and need. Some have questioned whether aggressive, and expensive, cancer treatments should be offered or provided to people of a certain age. This is a mistake. The law does not permit discrimination on the basis of age. Yet, with the changes in Medicare, some treatments may not be available to its beneficiaries (i.e., older adults). Medicare managed care, while purporting to expand benefits in terms of prescription drugs and eyeglasses, often limits the range of treatments for certain cancers. Typical is the limitation on treatment of prostate cancer. Some managed-care organizations offer only the transurethral resection of the prostate (TURP) even though it has significant side effects and risks and may not be the treatment of choice for everyone. This is an interesting inconsistency; while discrimination is against the law, the federal program of health care for older adults is able to specifically discriminate against them. Also important is to not make assumptions about what an "older" person may want. Simply because a patient with cancer is an older adult does not mean that he or she would not accept difficult treatments or make major lifestyle changes in order to improve his or her health. Therefore, all alternatives should be presented to patients so that they can choose from all possible options.

Elder-care specialists assert that age is a poor predictor of clinical success for medical treatment. Great variation exists among older adults in terms of how they respond to various therapies, including cancer therapies. Functional age—that is, the ability to perform activities of daily living—is a better predictor of health and ability to recover from illness than is chronological age (Ebersole & Hess, 1998). There is greater heterogeneity among elderly people than among younger people in many physiologic and psychological functions. Clearly, then, any cancer treatment decisions made on the basis of only chronological age are both unethical and legally actionable, as well as medically inappropriate.

Decision-making capacity: This concept originally was suggested by the President's Commission for the Study of Bioethical Problems in Medicine and Biomedical and Behavioral Research (1982), which provides for a presumption of *decision-making capacity* in adults. People who are elderly, "confused," mentally ill, or mentally retarded or who have been involuntarily committed to mental-health institutions do not automatically lose decision-making capacity; in each situation, an independent assessment of each person's ability to make decisions about healthcare treatment must be made.

When providing care to the older adult with cancer who may be depressed, experiencing the side effects of treatment, or consumed with fear, the nurse needs to carefully assess the patient's ability to make sound judgments. The nurse also must be alert to personal biases, as judgments made by one's patients may not be those the nurse would choose.

Decision-making capacity should not be confused with *competency*, which is a legal judgment rendered by a court determining whether a person is able to transact business or sign legally binding documents. Decision-making capacity may be determined by objective healthcare providers. The basis on which the assessment and determination were made must be documented in the patient's record.

Kind of cancer: For many people, particularly older adults, the pattern of managing health has been to not ask too many questions of healthcare providers. In their lifetime, the doctrine of informed consent has evolved to be very patient-oriented, but many older adults have not been able to take advantage of it. After hearing the word *cancer*, some people hear nothing else. Healthcare providers should make clear that different kinds of cancer in different stages have very different treatment outcomes. In some situations, it may be best to do nothing but watchful waiting. The elderly person may not be at risk by not undergoing treatment for cancers that are influenced by hormones. With the knowledge of the effect of nutrition, herbs, and vitamins on length and quality of life, advice on complementary and alternative therapies may be appropriate when other treatments are not contemplated. On the other hand, some cancers are very treatable and, with consent, should be treated aggressively.

Effectiveness of treatment: For some kinds of cancer, treatment may be only palliative. This must be made clear to the elderly patient. To choose therapies that may be difficult to manage and may only delay death while reducing the quality of remaining life may not be what the older person wants. However, clarity of possible outcomes is imperative for consent to be truly informed. Withholding, withdrawing, and refusing treatment are significant issues for nurses who are caring for older adults with cancer. There is a legal and ethical requirement to honor the refusal of treatments that a person does not want. Such treatments may be seen as disproportionately burdensome compared to the benefit that might be realized. Some treatments have a very remote chance of benefiting the person but may be tried to just "do something." The acts of withholding, withdrawing, and honoring refusal are ethically and legally permitted, even if the result is to hasten death. In fact, should the use of measures that relieve suffering and provide a greater measure of comfort result in death, healthcare providers generally are protected from prosecution for assisting with suicide. Daly (1995) suggested that nurses act in the patient's best interests by acting in accordance with patient values and choices, not the nurse's own. This way, when nurses are informed by family and friends of such values and choices, there is an obligation to accept them as long as no uncertainty about the patient's diagnosis and values exists.

Alternative and integrated approaches to cancer treatment: Healthcare institutions all over the United States are adding departments to their organizations that provide holistic, integrated therapies for patients who are receiving traditional medical treatment. Such treatments may be referred to as "alternative," although this refers to treatments used instead of conventional therapies; "complementary" is the more accurate term for therapies used in conjunction with conventional treatments. These new services are truly integrated, working closely with physicians and other providers to offer nutritional, herbal, touch, meditation, aroma, acupuncture, movement, and other therapies. These are available in addition to the typical cancer treatments of surgery, chemotherapy, and radiation therapy. Nurses are advised to educate themselves about complementary therapies and to integrate them for patients for whom they may be effective. This means performing a thorough assessment and providing objective, complete information about the therapies. Consultation with and referral to an alternative/complementary therapist is appropriate. Neglecting to provide such opportunities and information probably is not considered negligence, but it certainly is less than comprehensive, concerned care. Even if nurses are not convinced that such therapies are effective, patients should be provided with information and given a choice.

Nutrition and Hydration at the End of Life

Until recently, the issue of accepting or rejecting nutrition and hydration in end-of-life situations was not addressed in the law except to prohibit or prevent it. Now, however, many states have codified the rights of people to choose whether or not to have nutrition or hydration provided artificially. This usually is accomplished through an advance directive. When making decisions about nutrition and hydration or executing and implementing an advance directive, nurses may be guided by the patient's advance directives, the patient's or family's current choices, and the values expressed. Where advance directive laws explicitly address nutrition and hydration, patients may clearly and precisely express their wishes with regard to these treatments. The law seems to be moving toward preferring treatment limitation decisions to remain with the patient, perhaps through the advance directive. Nurses should be familiar with the laws about advance directives in the state where they are licensed or practice. Some laws distinguish between people who are terminally ill and those who would not otherwise die in the near future. The intention of the emerging law is that it is acceptable to allow a technologically preventable death to occur (Daly, 1995).

As long as a person has decision-making capacity, the advance directive is not needed. Of course, patients should not be advised to defer the execution of an advance directive until they "need it" because the time of its effectiveness may not be foreseeable. Patients may refuse food and fluids at any time. It is important that they understand what such refusal means physically, emotionally, and socially. Daly (1995) believed that advance directives are imperfect because they are expressions made in advance of situations that cannot be contemplated entirely. They are, however, the best protection of patient autonomy that is currently available.

When the word *artificially* is used, it usually means that nutrition and hydration are not ingested and absorbed in the usual manner. *Artificial* indicates use of a nasogastric, gastrostomy, or jejunostomy tube, often surgically implanted, or fluids provided intravenously or subcutaneously. The ANA (1992) issued a statement, originated by the Task Force on the Nurses Role in End-of-Life Decisions, concerning the issue of nurses finding a balance between the preservation of life and the facilitation of a dignified death. The ANA recognized the tensions that exist when caring for terminally ill patients and the consideration of intentionally hastening a patient's death as humane and compassionate. Yet, the traditional goals and values of the nursing profession mitigate against such actions. These issues need to be clarified in the minds of nurses who care for older adults with cancer because there are real considerations of treatment choices, imminent death, and other moral judgments. The ANA (1992) also asserted that artificial nutrition and hydration are different from the regular provision of food and water and may or may not be appropriate.

Wurzbach (1996) found that nurses who were morally certain about their values generally found that futile tube feedings were morally and esthetically repugnant and that their use diminished and violated the dignity of the dying person. Another issue that may need to be clarified is what "futility" actually means. Craig (1996) proposed that the simple and safe provision of minimal hydration may not be futile if it provides some comfort and help to the patient and calms the family's fears so that they can be reassured that the patient died of his disease and not from another ancillary cause.

Legal authorities recommend that nurses who are making or participating in decisions about withholding or withdrawing nutrition or hydration should rigorously consider the alternatives and the effects of each course of action. Additionally, the process and final decision should be carefully documented in the appropriate records. Nurses should determine, in advance of the need, the policies of the institution, who is consulted, and that the policies are clear and unambiguous. The institution's legal counsel is an excellent resource for explanation and interpretation of such policies.

Other issues regarding nutrition and hydration exist. This topic is far from being settled, either among legal authorities or healthcare providers. Some commentators believe that nutrition and hydration should be considered separately because they are quite different from each other. Nutrition often is not beneficial to terminally ill patients and, in fact, may be a significant burden, especially if surgical intervention is necessary. Hydration is a simpler process. It could be asserted that hydration is so simple that it could not legally be considered burdensome. The President's Commission (1982) and the U.S. Supreme Court supported the position that artificially provided nutrition and hydration are medical treatments that may be withheld or withdrawn from consenting patients or their families/surrogates. Families who wish to spare their loved ones such treatment often are accused of "starving the patient to death," even by healthcare providers. This rhetoric only serves to create profound guilt and conflict among families who are trying to provide for the patient's wishes. Nurses are well advised to clarify their own values before advising or commenting upon the families' decisions. Another point of view is espoused by Schiedermayer (1999), who asserted that withdrawal or withholding nutrition and hydration has the intent of causing death and is hard to justify.

Conclusion

Nurses who care for elderly patients with cancer must address many complex issues. Ethics and law meld at many points in the process. Change is the rule in terms of legal liability, ethical decision making, institutional policy, and treatment alternatives and possibilities. All of this affects oncology nursing practice. In the midst of change, knowledge is powerful—knowledge of standards and the efficacy of both traditional and nontraditional therapies. A comprehensive understanding of the elderly person with cancer in terms of values and expectations is imperative. Legal, ethical, spiritual, and medical variables have an impact on the care that one may choose to provide. Failure to be holistic, to consider all of the alternatives, and to individualize the patient's care may open the nurse up to legal action for negligence or some other violation of standards. Such failure is at least a deficiency of the caring that is central to nursing.

References

American Nurses Association. (1973). *Standards of nursing practice.* Kansas City, MO: American Nurses Publishing.

American Nurses Association. (1985). *Standards of nursing practice.* Washington, DC: American Nurses Publishing.

American Nurses Association. (1992). *Position statement: Foregoing nutrition and hydration* [Online]. Available: www.ana.org/readroom/position/ethics/etnutr.htm [1998, November].

American Nurses Association. (1995). *Standards and scope of gerontological nursing practice.* Washington, DC: American Nurses Publishing.

American Nurses Association & Oncology Nursing Society. (1996). *Statement on the scope and standards of oncology nursing practice.* Washington, DC: American Nurses Publishing.

Bandow, D., & Tanner, M. (1995, June 8). The wrong and right ways to reform medicare. *Policy Analysis, #230,* Washington, DC: Cato Institute.

Brown, J.G. (1995). *Medicare risk HMOs: Beneficiary enrollment and service access problems.* Washington, DC: U.S. Department of Health and Human Services, Office of Inspector General.

Canterbury v. Spence, 464 F.2d 772 (1972).

Craig, G.M. (1996). On withholding artificial hydration and nutrition from terminally ill sedated patients: The debate continues. *Journal of Medical Ethics, 22*(3), 147–153.

Daly, B.J. (1995). Withholding nutrition and hydration revisited. *Nursing Management, 26*(5), 30–39.

Ebersole, P., & Hess, P. (1998). *Toward health aging* (5th ed.). St. Louis: Mosby

Goodman, J.G., & Musgrave, G.L. (1992). *Patient power: Solving America's health care crisis.* Washington, DC: Cato Institute.

Meisel, A., & Kabnick, L.D. (1980). Informed consent to medical treatment: An analysis of recent legislation. 47. *University of Pittsburgh Law Review,* 407.

Natanson v. Kline, 350 P.2d 1093 (1960).

Patient Self-Determination Act, 42 U.S.C. 1395cc(f)(1), 43 U.S.C. 13396a(a) (Supp. 1991).

President's Commission for the Study of Bioethical Problems in Medicine and Biomedical and Behavioral Research. (1982). *Making health care decisions: The ethical and legal implications of informed consent in the patient-practitioner relationship.* Washington, DC: U.S. Government Printing Office.

Rosenblatt, R.E., Law, S.A., & Rosenbaum, S. (1997). *Law and the American health care system.* Westbury, NY: Foundation Press.

Schiedermayer, D.L. (1999). Why food and water are worth fighting about [Online]. Available: www.cmds.org/ethics/4_3_2a.htm [1999, September 3].

Trandel-Korenchuk, D.M., & Trandel-Korenchuk, K.M. (1997) *Nursing and the law* (5th ed.). Gaithersburg, MD: Aspen Publishers Inc.

Truman v. Thomas, 611 P.2d 902 (Cal. 1980).

Wurzbach, M.E. (1996). Long-term care nurses' ethical convictions about tube feeding. *Western Journal of Nursing Research, 18*(1), 63–76.

Index

Morbidity 1, 3, 9, 10, 15, 51, 59, 95, 101, 135

Mortality 1, 3, 5, 6, 9, 15, 17, 18, 51, 52, 56, 67, 95–97, 180

Mucinous carcinoma. *See* Breast cancer

Mucositis 44, 146–150

Mucous membranes 42, 43, 59, 64, 150

Myalgias 110

N

NANDA 103, 104, 105

National Cancer Institute (NCI) 1, 15, 17, 19, 28, 35, 68, 70, 71, 103

National Comprehensive Cancer Network (NCCN) 101

National Nursing Home Survey 6

Native Americans 4, 5, 86, 96

Nausea 16, 30, 42–44, 46, 55, 60, 62, 64, 81, 88–90, 92, 111, 115–117, 119, 121, 122, 129, 130–135, 145, 155

NCCN. *See* National Comprehensive Cancer Network (NCCN)

NCI. *See* National Cancer Institute (NCI)

Neoplasm 53, 55, 56

Neoplastic 9

Neurogenic pain 109

Neuropathy 60, 62

Neurotoxicities 60

Neutropenia 142, 148, 173

New Mexico 4, 5

Nolvadex. *See* Tamoxifen

Noninvasive 55, 87, 122, 124, 168

North American Nursing Diagnosis Association 174. *See* NANDA

Nucleic acid 19

Nurse practice acts 189, 190

Nursing home 107, 126, 174, 175. *See also* Long-term care setting

Nursing practice 126, 155, 177, 187, 189, 190, 195

Nutritional status 43, 64, 88, 90, 91, 146, 148

Nutritional supplements 89, 102

Nutritional support 43

O

Oncogenic 10

Oncology nursing practice 190, 195, 196

Opioids 118, 131, 139, 141, 142
side effects of 118

Osteoarthritis 21, 110

Osteoporosis 19, 21, 108, 110

P

Pacific Islanders 4, 6, 52

Pain 17, 20
assessment of 56, 110, 113
intensity scale 111, 113
management of 28, 41, 56, 77, 78, 111, 113, 115, 117, 119–122, 124–126, 168, 180

PAP. *See* Prostate-specific acid phosphatase (PAP)

Papillary carcinoma. *See* Breast cancer

Paraneoplastic pain syndrome (PPS) 110

Parenteral nutrition 45, 64, 145

Pathophysiology 30, 98, 130, 135, 142, 146

Peripheral nerve compression 109

Peripheral neuropathies 109, 110

Periurethral glands 97

Phantom limb pain (PLP) 109, 110

Planning 31–33, 37, 45, 88, 105

PLP. *See* Phantom limb pain (PLP)

PPS. *See* Paraneoplastic pain syndrome (PPS)

Presbyalgos 108

Prevention 7, 9–12, 14, 15, 17–19, 22, 43, 78, 79, 105, 138, 142, 146, 178

Procainamide derivative 134

Proliferation 71, 75, 90, 146

Prostate cancer 1–4, 6, 7, 12, 18, 51, 95–99, 101–105, 110, 121, 122, 126, 192

Prostate-specific acid phosphatase (PAP) 99, 101

Prostate-specific antigen (PSA) 18–20, 95, 97, 99–101, 190

PSA. *See* Prostate-specific antigen (PSA)

Q

Quality of life (QOL) 9, 10, 28, 30, 31, 61, 92, 95, 97, 105, 107, 108, 122, 131, 141, 142, 144, 146, 150, 153–155, 164, 168, 173, 175, 176, 178, 193

R

Radiation therapy 17, 18, 30, 43–45, 47, 52, 59, 61–65, 76–78, 81, 86, 88–91, 101, 104, 113, 120, 122, 133–136, 143, 146, 147, 173, 194
external beam 143
radioactive seed implant therapy 104

Radical prostatectomy 18, 101, 104, 105

Regulation 42, 189

Relaxation 42, 46, 123, 124, 135, 171

Renal 60, 114, 115

Retrograde ejaculation 105, 173

Risk factors 5, 9, 10, 11, 13, 15, 16, 18, 20, 53, 61, 67–70, 96, 146, 168, 171

RNA 19, 147

S

Screening 2, 9, 10, 15–22, 68, 69, 81, 85, 95–97, 99, 101, 106, 153, 190

Secondary prevention 10, 15, 24

Selective 5-HT$_3$ antagonist 134

Self-hypnosis 46, 123

Sexuality 16, 21, 28, 56, 64, 90, 96, 102, 105, 144, 165, 172–174

Sigmoidoscopy 19, 20

Skin 17, 59, 62–64, 78, 88, 90, 91, 102, 117, 139, 142

Smoking 11, 13, 14, 16, 52–54, 61, 80, 96, 105

Socioeconomic factors 96

Spiritual issues 31, 175, 178, 180, 182, 186

Standards of practice 189, 190

Stomach cancer 6

Supportive care 28, 29, 45

Supportive services 28

Supraclavicular node 57, 74

T

Tamoxifen 17, 18, 75, 76, 77, 81
Nolvadex 17
Zeneca Pharmaceuticals 17, 18

Thrombocytopenia 148

Tobacco 11, 13, 15, 52, 53, 54, 146

Total androgen ablation 101

Transrectal ultrasonography 95